MW00463628

Embodied
Healing

Embodied Healing

Survivor and Facilitator Voices from the Practice of Trauma-Sensitive Yoga

EDITED BY JENN TURNER

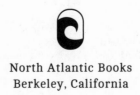

North Atlantic Books
Berkeley, California

Copyright © 2020 by Jenn Turner. All rights reserved. No portion of this book, except for brief review, may be reproduced, stored in a retrieval system, or transmitted in any form or by any means—electronic, mechanical, photocopying, recording, or otherwise—without the written permission of the publisher. For information contact North Atlantic Books.

Published by
North Atlantic Books
Berkeley, California

Cover art by Rob Johnson
Book design by Happenstance Type-O-Rama

Printed in the United States of America

Embodied Healing: Survivor and Facilitator Voices from the Practice of Trauma-Sensitive Yoga is sponsored and published by the Society for the Study of Native Arts and Sciences (dba North Atlantic Books), an educational nonprofit based in Berkeley, California, that collaborates with partners to develop cross-cultural perspectives, nurture holistic views of art, science, the humanities, and healing, and seed personal and global transformation by publishing work on the relationship of body, spirit, and nature.

North Atlantic Books' publications are available through most bookstores. For further information, visit our website at www.northatlanticbooks.com or call 800-733-3000.

This book contains material that may be triggering, including references to self-harm, eating disorders, sexual abuse, or trauma.

The following information is intended for general information purposes only. Individuals should always see their health care provider before administering any suggestions made in this book. Any application of the material set forth in the following pages is at the reader's discretion and is his or her sole responsibility.

Library of Congress Cataloging-in-Publication Data

Names: Turner, Jenn, editor.
Title: Embodied healing : survivor and facilitator voices from the practice
  of trauma-sensitive yoga / Jenn Turner, editor.
Description: Berkeley, California : North Atlantic Books, [2020] | Includes
  index. | Summary: "A collection of essays exploring the applications of
  TCTSY (Trauma Center Trauma Sensitive Yoga) as an evidence-based
  modality to help clients heal in the aftermath of trauma"—Provided by
  publisher.
Identifiers: LCCN 2020017363 (print) | LCCN 2020017364 (ebook) | ISBN
  9781623175344 (paperback) | ISBN 9781623175351 (ebook)
Subjects: LCSH: Psychic trauma—Physical therapy. | Yoga—Therapeutic use.
Classification: LCC RC552.T7 E43 2020 (print) | LCC RC552.T7 (ebook) |
  DDC 616.85/21—dc23
LC record available at https://lccn.loc.gov/2020017363
LC ebook record available at https://lccn.loc.gov/2020017364

1 2 3 4 5 6 7 8 9 KPC 24 23 22 21 20

This book includes recycled material and material from well-managed forests. North Atlantic Books is committed to the protection of our environment. We print on recycled paper whenever possible and partner with printers who strive to use environmentally responsible practices.

This book is dedicated to each survivor who has courageously taken a step into the unknown by joining us on our inquiry of how to reclaim embodiment in the aftermath of trauma; to my loving family, Ben, Annabel, and Emma, whose support for this project has been unwavering and steadfast; and to the wise, insightful, and dedicated contributors who made this book possible.

TABLE OF CONTENTS

FOREWORD

When you're breathing, when you're moving, when you open yourself up to
that new experience, there's something—I do believe that there's something
that is there. There's energy, there's mystery, there's connection, solidarity.
It's power . . . it adds another dimension to the healing in group. I see it,
I feel it—I do not know what the words exactly are, and I'm sure there are
words that could describe it more. There's something vulnerable about it
too, there's that connection in our vulnerability that can be pretty powerful.

—Trauma-sensitive yoga research participant, excerpted from Nguyen-Feng
et al. (2019) Spirituality in Clinical Practice article

I REMEMBER THE EXACT MOMENT when I first heard of trauma-sensitive yoga. Even now, I remain in awe and appreciation of the seemingly serendipitous, intertwining paths that led me to it. Shortly after making the move halfway across the country for my counseling psychology doctoral studies, I decided to participate in a local women's health conference hosted by the University of Minnesota. I'm not sure what compelled me to take on such a task two weeks into a new city and program, but that is one part of the serendipity.

At the conference, I presented a poster on a very small pilot study that I had conducted on yoga and prenatal health perceptions. I only pursued this pilot study because the researcher for whom I previously worked (Dr. James Blando, Old Dominion University/Eastern Virginia Medical School) suggested that I start a yoga project. This was definitely far from the scope of his community and environmental health lab. But because of the time I had put into the lab, he was simply extending a generous opportunity to support me on an outside project related to a known interest of mine. I hadn't even considered conducting research on something that I viewed as a non-academic practice, but I took on the task. And so, that is how I ended up at the women's health conference.

Standing forlornly in front of my poster that was solitarily situated at the endcap of an aisle (I'm sure many researchers can relate!), I shyly smiled at an individual who was meandering around the space. She kindly paused to read my poster and asked me about my next steps in the presented project. I informed her that the yoga research was simply a side project, as I was refocusing my research on inter-personal trauma. In turn, she casually informed me that her public health colleague at the university, Dr. Cari Jo Clark, was integrating these two areas in a trauma-sensitive yoga study. And that was the exact moment when I first heard of trauma-sensitive yoga.

Fast forwarding a bit, I connected with the wonderful folks at the Domestic Abuse Project, a community-based nonprofit agency located in Minneapolis, as well as Dr. Cari Jo Clark, who is now at Emory University, and David Emerson, who at the time had recently coauthored his first book, *Overcoming Trauma through Yoga: Reclaiming Your Body*, which I held in the highest regard. I held it in such regard that I can recall myself sitting in the 717 Delaware Building on campus while holding the unopened book with the utmost care and eagerness. The message of Trauma Center Trauma-Sensitive Yoga (TCTSY) resonated with my whole being—my body and my mind, my belief in the inextricable link between mental and physical wellness, and my belief that our bodies in the present hold our pains from the past. Collabora-tion with this inspirational team culminated in the first feasibility study of TCTSY, which was published in *Complementary Therapies in Clinical Practice* in 2014. My research line on mind-body trauma care was taking root.

The impacts of trauma-sensitive yoga can be difficult to express in words, as the effects are simply and truly felt, deeply and internally.

The idea of embodiment, of connecting to our inward wisdom and experiences, intrinsically implies a wordlessness in understanding oneself on such a level. As one research participant recounted to me in regard to her trauma-sensitive yoga experience: "There's energy, there's mystery, there's connection, solidarity. It's power . . . it adds another dimension to the healing in group. I see it, I feel it—I do not know what the words exactly are, and I'm sure there are words that could describe it more."

Jenn Turner skillfully takes on that challenge. The book that you are holding in your hands contains spoken and unspoken treasures, explicit words and implicit feelings. You are holding a collection of stories that have not been so viscerally told altogether at any point in this world. These are narratives of resilience, of individuals reentering their bodies following the aftermath of trauma and of individuals supporting others in reentering and refriending their bodies. To me, reading *Embodied Healing* is like embarking on a journey with each student and each facilitator, in which I feel greatly humbled to receive their honest and sharing spirit. I can only hope that you feel similarly.

Like when I held *Overcoming Trauma through Yoga* in my hands for the first time, the first time I opened the manuscript of *Embodied Healing* brought up a reverent reaction in me. I could not help but feel immense gratitude for the privilege of reading this work and toward all of the diverse voices represented in it, the first of surely many future books by the well-versed Jenn Turner, editor extraordinaire and more. For instance, Jenn also serves as the Justice Resource Institute's Center for Trauma and Embodiment (CFTE) co-founder alongside David Emerson, CFTE's director of training, TCTSY's program coordinator, and a trauma-informed therapist in private practice. With knowledge gained from these roles, Jenn has been able to collate stories and craft them in an order that firmly builds upon itself and TCTSY themes: sharing authentic experiences, making choices, cultivating present-moment awareness, and taking effective action. May each participant's story, each of which is represented in a fully individualized chapter, allow you to engage with these themes as well.

I invite you to now reflect on the paths that led you to hold *Embodied Healing* in your hands at this time. You may notice that there is no one path, but rather, an entwinement of paths that have crossed into this very instance of you reading these words. If you'd like, take in a breath and take in this moment. This is the moment before you take in the narratives on the following pages. Who knows where these narratives will take you. Two decades ago, I curiously took out a dusty yoga VHS I found in my childhood home; little did I know that my exploratory practice back then would eventually lead me to where I am today. Seemingly serendipitous paths are indeed intertwined. Our lives comprise points of connection, within ourselves and with each other, with our bodies and minds operating in tandem. The stories before you might simultaneously take you somewhere yet nowhere, rightfully into the inner essence of yourself. We as human beings are inherently united in our felt experiences. The stories in your hands belong to the students and the facilitators—the storywriters. And they, too, belong to you.

Viann N. Nguyen-Feng, PhD, MPH, RYT

Director of the Mind-Body Trauma Care Lab,
Department of Psychology, University of Minnesota,
Duluth

INTRODUCTION

Jenn Turner

HOW CAN WE DEFINE *TRAUMA?* Is it about the severity of the transgression? The duration of violation or omission? When it happens during lifespan? Groups ranging from the National Child Traumatic Stress Network to the American Psychological Association all define a traumatic event by the type of action that occurs, such as violence, neglect, or natural disaster. Understanding what can cause traumatic responses may be helpful in many contexts—but when we focus on *what* happened, we unknowingly participate in a cycle of invalidating survivors' experiences.

Trauma should be defined by the person who experiences it, not by an expert or external force. Many trauma survivors have endured the pain of an expert or provider telling them that what they experienced could not have led to post-traumatic stress disorder (PTSD) or complex trauma; or that perhaps what they experienced was a "little t" trauma. This kind of power imbalance further induces shame, self-blame, and isolation. Trauma should be understood by the survivor's experience. Trauma should be understood in how it leaves its mark, often for a lifetime, scorched into the brains and bodies of those who experience it.

What is it like to live in a body that has experienced complex trauma, repeated trauma that happens within a relationship and over the span of time? What is it like to be connected to other humans when the core of complex trauma is relational betrayal? These are questions I have been exploring through the lens of Trauma Center Trauma-Sensitive Yoga (TCTSY), along with my colleague David Emerson, for almost two decades. Through research, focus groups, participant feedback, trainings, and collectively leading thousands of TCTSY sessions, we have learned that the impact of complex trauma can be both profound and debilitating, and that the care given must reflect this impact.

Traumatic experiences become deeply embedded in our muscles, organs, and bones. It is not only that the body remembers[1] but that the trauma still lives in the body. Traumatic memories are at their core both timeless and somatic in nature. As they play over and over in the mind and body, these memories become intertwined in calibrating a host of automatic processes—impacting the rate and depth of breath, how the autonomic nervous system regulates the heartbeat, or how the immune system functions, to name a few. There is also evidence that the brain struggles to distinguish between past and present when traumatic memories and content become triggered. This can lead to the felt experiences that trauma is happening right here, right now. Trauma responses become more entrenched as memories and experiences replay over and over again, reinforcing our protective defenses, many of which are held in our bodies.

These physical manifestations provide concrete evidence to a survivor that bad experiences don't end; they continue to be very much alive and ongoing. The impact of trauma on the body can range from intangible to palpable. Over time the physical consequences are measurable and severe. The Adverse Childhood Experiences study has found an association between trauma and risk of heart disease, stroke, and cancer. Patients who reported six or more adverse experiences had a nearly twenty-year reduction in life expectancy.[2] This study gives us concrete evidence of what survivors and providers have always known: Trauma changes us. It changes our minds and bodies.

Understanding how the echoes of trauma continue to reverberate in the body led David and me (and many more folks) to wonder about the lived, somatic experience of a trauma survivor.

For example, what is it like to inhabit a body that was invisible in a family or relationship? In some families and relationships, a survivor's body simply occupying space might have been enough to enrage a parent or partner into violence, manipulation, or utter rejection. Ongoing abusive dynamics like this can lead to a detachment or a disembodied relationship to one's own body.

Some of our participants have shared having the experience of looking at their own hands or feet and feeling that they didn't belong to them, or feeling the touch of their own hand on their leg or arm feel like the hand of a stranger. I use this example not to illustrate something moral—in fact, for many survivors of trauma, disconnecting from their felt experience may have been a display of the human organism's brilliance: What better way to remove ourselves from the reality of our body than to largely feel like we don't have one? While it's entirely possible to live a life where we feel detached or removed from our body, it may also be true that at some point living in this way becomes limiting or difficult.

What is it like to live in a body that was coerced, shamed, or neglected by a loved one? A participant in our randomized control trial concisely articulated the impact:

Sometimes I feel triggered, it was like somebody else used this body and it doesn't feel good, and I will never feel good.[3]

When a person takes another's body through physical or psychological force, the victim can feel a horrific loss of power and agency. Survivors may find themselves rejecting or loathing their body, which can in turn make it utterly impossible to care for or listen to a body that was such a profound liability. This again may be a remarkably adaptive way to coexist with a body that is an "implicit reminder that accompanied the terror of trauma."[4]

In the words of neuroscientist Antonio Damasio, "There is no such thing as a disembodied mind. The mind is implanted in the brain, and the brain is implanted in the body."[5] Despite mountains of evidence that the body and the brain are inextricably linked, and in particular in the aftermath of trauma, the primary modalities of therapeutic intervention in the Western medical model predominately involve *thinking and talking* about what has happened. In fact, trauma-focused cognitive behavioral therapy, which implores clients to change their thinking or narrative about what has happened through talking and writing, is considered to be the gold standard in treating trauma. A close second is exposure therapy, asking clients to desensitize to triggers of their trauma—despite our knowledge of how trauma over-activates and enlarges the amygdala, the part of the brain responsible for mediating our fear response.

Unfortunately, many clients in traditional therapy report getting stuck, or worse, repeatedly triggered as they recount experiences of trauma and are asked to increase their tolerance of these horrific events. Somatic approaches to healing, such as somatic experiencing and sensorimotor psychotherapy, have been educating practitioners and survivors of trauma about how to bring the body into traditional talk-therapy settings. These approaches, and others, seek to integrate the body by thinking, moving, and talking to address what has happened and how the body may be affected today by what occurred in the past. Research has also indicated that the more a survivor becomes triggered, the less they are able to speak about their experience. Brain imaging shows us that as the brain's fear center is activated, its narrative area becomes de-emphasized, making language much less accessible. Which leads to another question: Do we need to talk about what has happened in order to make meaning of the past?

The purpose of this book is to share with treatment practitioners and survivors of trauma what it might look like to create conditions for processing and holding experiences of trauma *without* talking about them. To hold a space where survivors could show up, exactly as they are, and explore having a body, noticing their body, and possibly making choices in that body without needing to find language to explain or articulate what is happening. Trauma Center Trauma-Sensitive Yoga (TCTSY) has proven to be one way of exploring this type of trauma healing. Through dismantling power dynamics and recognizing that there is no prescriptive way to heal from trauma, we have developed and tested a way to practice yoga that works to honor the unique wisdom within each survivor. How trauma both is experienced by the survivor and manifests are unequivocally unique; therefore, healing must also be equally as individualized. I am not suggesting that TCTSY be a stand-alone treatment. There is deep value in finding language for what has happened in the wake of trauma, but sometimes there are no words. When survivors are continually asked to speak about an experience they may not have words for, frustration and re-traumatization may be unintended outcomes. When trauma is wordless, instead of trying to talk about it, we need to *move about it.*

I have often been asked "Why yoga? Why not Trauma-Sensitive Tai Chi or Spinning?" I can confidently answer only the first question. We chose to explore yoga as an adjunctive treatment for trauma for many reasons. The contemplative and physical practices associated with yoga have a history spanning thousands of years, stemming from a particular geographical and sociocultural milieu (present-day India and Pakistan) but spreading into every corner of the globe. Acknowledging and committing ourselves to some of the deepest roots of these practices provided critical foundations that we felt were specifically aligned to the requirements of trauma healing, such as ahimsa, the deep practice of non-harming, and svadhyaya, the practice of self-study. Yoga in the West, and the United States in particular, has become widely popular and therefore available to many . . . but, as we have learned through our work, it is not welcoming or available to all. Although this book doesn't specifically explore the harm done by colonization and the commodification of yoga, both of which are deeply important for us as practitioners to explore and study, we as a community are striving to honor the roots of yoga and, in so doing, make yoga available to people who might not always feel welcome or safe.

This book is divided into sections based on themes that we have found essential in creating conditions for safely, ethically, and holistically engaging in body-based trauma treatment. These themes can provide anchors in the often-choppy waters of body-based trauma recovery.

Shared Authentic Experience

The majority of trauma is perpetrated by someone who is known, trusted, or even loved by the victim, and a natural outcome is that relationships can become triggering and overwhelming. Pioneer and visionary Judith Herman writes, "The core experiences of trauma are disempowerment and disconnection from others."[6] With disconnection at the core of trauma, many survivors face families, friends, and a world at large that seek to silence, deny, or rewrite their experience. It's no wonder that trusting others and sharing in experiences can be challenging. When we start to work with a survivor, from the very first interaction, we attend to the relationship. Without building a relationship where power is shared and the internalized structure of expert versus client (or abuser versus victim) is dismantled, the practice of trauma-sensitive yoga becomes just another pill to swallow. Making choices, being embodied in the present, and taking action are meaningful because they happen within a relationship where a survivor is met and known, with respect, curiosity, and transparency on the part of the facilitator.

Making Choices

There is an overpowering loss of choice at the heart of all trauma. An experience might range from being trapped in a family or relationship, being physically held down, or being born into an identity that is oppressed by the dominant culture. For a survivor who is triggered by sensations within their body—for example, the experience of sensing their own heartbeat—they may begin to become less physically active in order to keep their heart rate down. Perhaps they're doing less of what they enjoy and becoming more socially isolated, leading to a lowered sense of self and a loss of relationships. In the cascading impact of trauma, we see over time how adaptive patterns of coping become entrenched, and life begins to have fewer and fewer choices.

When I do talk therapy with clients, we plan for choices, and we think about choices that could be made in the future. With TCTSY we are inviting people to practice making choices, in the moment, right now. So many of our clients talk about how they feel like they can't change things: "Things are always going to be this way." What is it like for people to actually feel themselves make a choice in the yoga session, to make a choice in their body based on what they feel? It appears that making choices in the moment, within a relationship, can have a ripple effect far beyond any individual moment. We will attempt to illustrate the significance of what it means to make choices in this way.

Present Moment

For many trauma survivors, one of the challenges they face is living in a body where the trauma continues to feel like it is still happening, in a brain/body that cannot always distinguish between past and present when triggered. It's not the idea that the trauma is happening but the embodied sense that it is. This may breed shame, embarrassment, or frustration for the survivor whose body generates a startle response, sweat, or constriction during what they may have expected to be a relaxing walk at the beach or a social outing with friends. Through the lens of TCTSY we aim to invite the exploration of the present moment through mindful movement. As facilitator and participant move together, opportunities to cultivate interoception (the awareness of what we feel within our bodies) are offered, and in those moments when our physical and neurophysiological reality align, we are present. And that moment, however brief, is *not* trauma.

In this section we hope to demonstrate how with TCTSY we offer opportunities for survivor and facilitator to share in an experience where the goal is not to perfect a yoga form or even to self-regulate. In our work yoga serves as a tool for people to explore doing something together that can actually look quite different from each other on the outside, yet we are still exploring connection together. We as facilitators take ownership of our own experience, and participants are encouraged and supported to take ownership of theirs.

Effective Action

The experience of trauma often involves being physically held down—immobilized. This could mean being stuck under a car, restrained by an assailant, or strapped or tied down. It also might include being trapped in an abusive relationship or dynamic for any number of reasons. Not only does this lead to a lack of choice as mentioned earlier, but it can also engender a deep sense of ineffectiveness within our organism, sometimes called learned helplessness. This is a way in which trauma can lead to a loss of agency. We may have learned that we don't have the ability to change our circumstances, our emotional state, or how our body feels. When we bring the body into trauma treatment, we can offer opportunities to practice effectiveness through movement. In the context of TCTSY this can look like adjusting our body position when experiencing unwanted sensation, or this might mean walking to the front of the room to get a prop to assist with a form. What has been so compelling is learning the ways that this has translated "off the mat" for so many of our participants.

The final pillar of our work is non-coercion. This has not been divided into its own section, because it is a constant in all our work. Far too often, providers are guilty of benevolent coercion—sometimes subtly, oftentimes not so—coercing clients into doing what the provider thinks will help the client, or make them better, or heal them. This behavior can appear kind or nurturing on the outside, but it ultimately usurps the survivor's ability to claim agency of their own healing journey, however circuitous or maladaptive it may appear through the lens of pathology. In this work, and all trauma work, we believe that the survivor has a right to dignity through claiming their own choice to engage in treatment, or not. You will read us struggling with this and working to find ways to offer agency and empowerment in structures and environments that don't always support that.

Each chapter in the book aims to provide a glimpse into the process, as best articulated by a participant:

I reclaimed my body. That is a gift because I so hated my body. Or claimed it, not reclaimed it, because I was so young. I claimed it. It was a long process to consider myself not an outline . . . I think yoga helped define. Just inhabiting my own skin is a major step forward.[7]

Each client was consulted throughout the writing process and sometimes contributed their own words. Some chapters are written by yoga participants and others by facilitators who are also survivors of trauma. Some chapters are written in delicate collaboration, where voices of facilitator and participant are intertwined. I would invite you to notice the dance between facilitator and survivor in building a relationship. When relationships may have been the very scene of the trauma or crime, it takes extra care to create one that is safe enough to do this delicate, deep, and sometimes painful work.

When someone has experienced the underbelly of humanity, seeing and experiencing people at their very worst, to witness the transformation that can take place when the body is re-inhabited is simply breathtaking. I hope that this collection of stories from the practice provides a window into what healing from trauma can look like from a body-forward perspective.

SHARED AUTHENTIC EXPERIENCE

The Relationship Comes First

Building a Container for Embodied Work

Jenn Turner

AUDREY FIRST BEGAN WORKING WITH me doing one-on-one yoga. I prepared for our first session by reflecting on the core aspect: working with trauma is relational. It doesn't matter if you are working through a somatic, artistic, analytical, or medical lens—the relationship comes first. When trauma happens in families, intimate partnerships, and close connections, the relationship is the scene of the crime. It is within the relationship that the betrayal happened. Trauma is most often not random but rather deeply personal. When we invite clients to engage with us as caregivers, they are returning to the crime scene. Asking survivors to trust or rely on our judgment, or our plan for healing when they have been so deeply betrayed within relationships, is asking for the impossible. The only way to meet this is to not ask or expect survivors to trust us. I prepared for my first individual yoga session with Audrey by working on letting go—surrendering any sense of expertise or mastery about how to heal trauma or what might be helpful to her. This gave me the mental and emotional space to get curious about how to co-create connection and healing with Audrey.

I knew very few details about Audrey's history at our first meeting. What I did know was that her history of trauma and poor outcomes in traditional mental health treatment led her to seek an embodied approach. I was attuned to her body language as I sought to accommodate her and make her feel as welcome as possible. Audrey seemed hesitant. She walked in with her shoulders drawn down, gaze low with only fleeting glances toward my eyes. She seemed to hold her body as if to not occupy space.

We made our way to the yoga space, a conference room that moonlights as a studio after the clearing of chairs, closing of blinds, and changing of lighting. As we got acquainted, I noticed she looked down as she spoke softly. When we began to work out how to set up our yoga mats, her voice became more steady, more self-assured, as she expressed how she wanted to position her body in relation to mine. She chose to roll out her mat, so we created an L shape. This allowed her to look at me and follow along, if she chose, while also offering privacy and perhaps a sense that I would not be watching or critiquing her. In the context of TCTSY, navigating how to position our bodies in relation to one another is not an insignificant task. To create safety, it is imperative that the yoga facilitator gives the student as much physical space as the student wants, given the confines, in an effort to not startle or trigger the student with their body. This was also our first opportunity, of many more to come, navigating how to be in relation to one another.

Before beginning to work with yoga forms, Audrey and I sat and talked a little about what she might expect during our hour-long session. When starting to engage in the collaborative work of trauma-sensitive yoga, one important point to negotiate is how the student will communicate when something doesn't feel safe in their body or if they need to alter the yoga forms or to stop. In one-on-one yoga sessions of any kind, the facilitator typically does most of the talking while the student is largely quiet. In TCTSY we aim to create an environment where the student has a voice in as many ways as possible, both within the session and around it. This may involve the use of email or anonymous surveys as well as an invitation for feedback during and at the end of a session. It can be especially difficult for survivors to give voice to their experiences. Part of the betrayal of trauma is that the victim's needs, desires, or wishes are ignored or irrelevant to perpetrators. Communicating about how the process is and isn't working becomes central to the work. To support Audrey in taking the risk to voice her needs, we found various ways for her to communicate. It was even more important that I met her in this with my own openness and honesty to hearing her feedback.

When I asked Audrey how we might negotiate this together, she said something I have often heard from survivors of interpersonal trauma: "It's hard for me to say something in these kinds of situations."

Audrey was trying to tell me that expressing when something didn't feel okay was difficult. Whether talking to a therapist, yoga teacher, loved one, or stranger, speaking up was hard, if not nearly impossible.

I replied, "Is there some other way you might let me know that something isn't feeling right to you? Maybe tapping your finger on the mat, flipping over a piece of paper, or moving into a specific form?"

She responded after a brief pause, "I am not sure. I sometimes don't know if something doesn't feel okay until later."

This brief moment highlights one of the fundamental challenges of inviting survivors to make choices with their body. In acts of sexual or physical violence, both of which I later learned Audrey had experienced, a perpetrator makes a certain claim on a victim's body, insinuates and usurps control, and then proceeds to make choices about that body based on *their* motivations. If you are the victim, in that moment your body is no longer your own. Many find themselves detaching from their experience, and therefore their body, to simply survive. Through our continued work I learned how skillfully Audrey had learned to ignore or mute cues from her body in order to keep herself safe.

Repeated experiences and replaying traumatic memories compound the impacts leading to complex trauma. The continued assault of memories usurps the ability to have agency over what happens to, or with, the very body they inhabit. Over time the pattern of detachment or alienation from one's own body is deepened and solidified. This mechanism of selective disembodiment is quite adaptive and brilliant; it's a survival tool. When your body becomes a little less your own, it becomes possible for you to live through the fracturing experience of someone enacting their will upon you. If you have had to tolerate intense and/or repeated overwhelming sensations within your body, there may be a dulling of sensation altogether. Many times there is a fracturing of sensation as well, where parts of you hold the physical and/or emotional pain of the overwhelming experience.

This is a way of surviving the terror of physical or sexual trauma, but it may also lead to disconnection from a wide range of bodily sensations including pain, discomfort, or pleasure. On the one hand there is survival, but on the other, what is life without reliable access to one's embodied experience? Once the danger of trauma has passed, our body is left imprinted with the unique ability to disconnect, to turn off and tune out our somatic experience. Living life without access to physical pain, pleasure, or other sensations becomes a difficult way to live life.

After a brief check-in, I typically start each individual session with twenty minutes of yoga seated on the mat or in a chair. First I invite students to begin to bring awareness into their bodies through movement, followed by interoception, the act of bringing conscious awareness to sensation within our own body, and finally awareness of breath. Audrey often found this a useful way to start. After orienting to her physical experience by thinning the veil of detachment, we typically paused to speak about anything she may have noticed in her body and if she would like the session to move in a particular direction. Sometimes Audrey would ask for a more energetic series of postures; other times she might direct us to stay grounded on the mat. This was typically a collaborative process that also included her sometimes asking me to lead, with the caveat that she would let me know if she needed something different.

At this point in one of our early sessions, Audrey spoke about how hearing me cuing to notice her breath was challenging. Again I heard that strength in her voice that briefly appeared in our very first meeting. She appeared to have found clarity that interacting with her breathing and tolerating the feeling or sound of her own breath was overwhelming. We decided that I would not cue breath for the rest of the session. In that same moment, she articulated that it was helpful to her when I invited her to notice feeling in a specific part of her body within the yoga forms.

In this exchange, Audrey was able to use her voice. The student-teacher or client-provider relationship inherently brings an imbalance of power, which if not carefully attended to can mirror trauma dynamics. A safe therapeutic relationship hinges on the facilitator's willingness to listen and modify the yoga session based on the student's needs. Which also means letting go of the belief that we, as the providers, are the experts.

I believe this was a poignant moment in building a foundation for Audrey to be supported by another in making choices based solely on her internal experience. In the therapeutic world, providers often find themselves pushing an agenda, however well intentioned, of coercing their client to breathe differently, calm their nervous system, or change their relationship to their body based on the provider's expectations. Supporting Audrey's preference to not focus on her breathing required me to let go of my attachment to outcomes for her. Despite my knowing all the ways that focusing on breath and changing breathing patterns could have positive impacts, *for Audrey* it was overwhelming and unhelpful. Both the yoga and the therapeutic worlds have sets of beliefs about how a client should heal from trauma, but in truth healing must be survivor-led. In my experience, for healing to occur, Audrey, like most of my clients, had to find agency within her self. With my support, Audrey was able to make choices about what felt safe and most available in *her* body, thereby taking an important step toward agency.

Each individual session typically ends with some sort of seated yoga, followed by an opportunity to interact with rest and stillness. Sarah, a survivor of complex intergenerational trauma, tried in our early sessions to rest on her back, as is often expected at the end of a yoga class, but found it very difficult. Sarah had first started coming to the drop-in group classes, where she hoped that community and body-based experiences would provide a welcome support to her talk therapy. She found that being in a group was more challenging than expected due to the unpredictability of participants in the room and the pressure that she was putting on herself to build relationships with other participants. We transitioned for several months to weekly individual sessions.

Resting and stillness are vulnerable positions for many survivors of trauma. When the body slows, it can create an opening for physiological anxiety and mental demons, sabotaging any attempts at being at ease in one's body. I have found it useful to offer survivors a wide range of choices at this point in the practice. In this work, we meet many of our students in a state of high alert that makes stillness or calm an incongruent experience. Feeling peacefulness in a yoga class isn't a given, nor is it required, for that matter. For a trauma survivor, time, consistency, and choice, within the context of a safe enough relationship, are needed to create the potential for stillness or peace.

Sarah discovered that it was dangerous being on her back in stillness after an hour's practice—she had just spent more time noticing her body and witnessing felt sensation than she might have previously spent in a whole week. As Sarah turned toward the sensory experience of her own body, she found it harder to keep painful and traumatic memories at bay. Sometimes there would be a flood of chaotic traumatic content during the rest.

Herein lies one of the powerful choice-points that we face in TCTSY: Do we turn toward somatic memories and unearth trauma that has been stuck or stored? Or do we turn away from these sometimes-catastrophic memories in favor of stability and being present in the moment? This is a culmination of several aspects of TCTSY that we hope to explore in the coming sections of this book. No choice is right for everyone. Some survivors may find they want to turn toward painful memories for a whole host of reasons: knowing what happened, resolving confusion, not keeping secrets. Others may decide they don't want to turn toward a memory because they cannot change the past or the risk of being haunted by what might be disturbing traumatic content is too great.

Sarah and I had slowly built a relationship where, she later shared, she didn't feel like she needed to please me, or succeed at yoga, or be "strong enough" to face her demons. She could just be, and for her that meant she could turn away from traumatic memories and keep them compartmentalized.

One of the goals of trauma treatment in my experience is supporting clients and participants in being self-led. Moments like this test that. Should Sarah turn toward these memories? Would she feel relief if she did? Am I letting her down as a provider by supporting her in compartmentalizing? I turned these questions over and over in my mind but always came back trusting that Sarah, not I, had the wisdom we needed to follow.

After working together with Audrey for a few months, at the end of a session I asked if there was anything she observed about her practice that she wanted to share. She paused and took a breath. "I am starting to understand that there is no 'right' way to do things here." I nodded in support. She continued, "Which is no small thing, given the home I grew up in. Where I grew up there was a clear right and wrong way to do things. If you didn't do things the right way . . . there were consequences, severe consequences."

It was stunning to hear this from her, as one of the powerful ways trauma takes root in the lives of survivors is through creating a lack of choice or options. With TCTSY we explore this lack of choice as it relates to the body. Perpetrators of trauma often become hyper-vigilant toward the bodies of their victims. Perpetrators attune to the bodies around them in order to know better how to impose power and control over them. On a cellular level, survivors learn to move, breathe, and express feelings in a very specific way to avoid being noticed or to please the perpetrator in order to minimize, as best as possible, experiences of pain or violence.

Over time as Audrey and I explored her discovery of choices, she came to another realization. One day she said, "I am noticing that I have been living my whole life as if I have no choice or say in things. What we are doing here is making me think I have to completely change the way I am living my life . . . but I have no idea how to do that." We paused for a moment to take in the gravity of her words.

I found myself immediately becoming overwhelmed by what it might feel like for her to consider overhauling her life in this way. I spoke first: "It's remarkable that you are making these connec-tions from the work we are doing. One way you could approach the idea of making changes in your life is to continue to show up here and to practice making choices in your body." She nodded in agreement, so I continued: "And it seems that what is happening in our yoga sessions has been filtering off the mat and into your daily life. I wonder if we can allow that to continue to happen and changes may just occur organically?" Audrey nodded in agreement and looked at me: "That feels right."

In that moment, we could have gotten lost in the weeds, so to speak. We might have started planning and analyzing how she could make changes in her life. I could easily have shifted into a more directive role and given her "homework" to try to manifest more change in her life. This would have led us down a path fur-ther and further away from her experience in her body, as it was unfolding in the moment, and the truth is that she was already making changes; they were already happening. This also would have undermined power sharing and our shared authentic experience that was making these choices so meaningful. Audrey was making choices in close relationship with me, and I wasn't pushing her to get "better" more quickly or asking her to conform to my idea of healing.

In the months to follow, Audrey shifted from individual sessions to my group class. She continued to explore making choices in her body based on her experience but now in a community of other survivors. At this time she also began seeing me for private psychotherapy.

One evening I noticed her moving differently from my cues throughout much of class. When I led the class through standing forms, she chose to sit on her mat and move into forward folds. She chose to move onto her back while I offered movement in seated. When I witness moments like this, it feels like a significant milestone. A student, within the context of her peers and facilitator, being able to listen to signals from her body and make choices that are different from what the group is doing, is extraordinary. Making choices in this way is also fraught. As Audrey had articulated months before, she had learned as a child that there were profoundly right and wrong choices. Making wrong choices in her family had resulted in severe consequences.

In TCTSY we invite clients to be in relationship with us and fellow students by highlighting that we can each make different choices about what we do on our mats and with our bodies while still being in community with one another. This is the opposite of the trauma paradigm. Trauma in families and systems demands conformity. Victims are forced to assimilate to belief systems, rules, and rituals that often erase individuality and identity. In cultivating a shared relationship, we can celebrate and name our differences, building connection through those differences.

I saw Audrey in my office the day after the class where she had made so many choices, and we spoke about what she had experienced in class the evening before. I said, "I noticed that it seemed like you were listening to your body and making choices last night, and I was wondering what that was like for you?" Audrey immediately responded, "I was sure that after class, when I confirmed our time for today, you would say no. That you would be angry and disappointed that I wasn't doing the postures everyone else was doing. That somehow I was so awful for having done that you wouldn't want to see me in your office or ever come back to class. I was really surprised when you confirmed our time and didn't seem upset or angry."

Audrey's words confirmed what I had also experienced with Sarah. As yoga teachers and therapists, if we want to help our clients listen to their inner voice, to be self-led, we cannot have ulterior motives to control or manipulate their bodies or actions, however well meaning. When we find ourselves wanting our clients to use their breath to better regulate or find ways to ground themselves more efficiently, however kind our intentions are, we must check out these intentions.

When someone has experienced repeated relational trauma, their capacity for sensing frustration, annoyance, or irritation from others is remarkable. This is about survival. They are at the scene of the crime. Relationships are where bad things happen, and as a result they become a liability. Therefore, people are a liability. Frustration, annoyance, and irritation can quickly shift into anger or rage. Survivors know that, sense that. If I bring traces of annoyance to a student who is moving however she wants on her mat, she will feel and experience that as danger. If I push for someone to turn toward traumatic content, even if their body is saying no, that is a reenactment of trauma.

To move toward safety in the relationship, I have to truly surrender my desire to have my class move in rhythm with me. This surrender becomes embodied. I cannot simply tell participants that they can make choices; I have to show them by greeting the lack of synchronicity in the room with warmth and readiness. It is an ongoing process of letting go of my attachment to the benefits of a specific yoga form or breathing pattern, or of "my way." It is an ongoing practice of letting go of seeing myself as the expert and allowing the survivor to claim her own expertise. It is a continual practice to step out of the way and allow each survivor to find her unique path to a safe relationship with her body and self.

Connecting in Safety

Waking Up to the Reality of Interconnectedness and Learning to Tolerate It through Facilitation

Kirsten Voris

MY MEMORIES OF BEING SMALL are few and far between. They are islands floating in a sea of what I think of as body knowledge—a sense of things. I remember impressions, mostly. There are no words or stories attached to them.

By the time I started grade school I was an insomniac with chronic headaches. Long before that, I had internalized a sense of my role and my value. I knew that if I was struggling or experiencing a feeling, that if someone was angry or disappointed, it was my job to fix it. If I couldn't fix it, I had to figure out how to handle it.

For most of my life I've discounted my own preferences because it seemed irrelevant to my primary project—feeling safe. I learned to hang back and wait, to see which way the wind was blowing. I chose what I thought others wanted me to choose. I was good at making myself small and, once I was a teenager, even better at making myself scarce. Being smart was important in my family. Being funny, if timed right, could earn smiles and laughter. I learned to deploy these strategies, and they became part of my armor.

Feeling lovable, I sensed, was a matter of getting things right. There seemed to be ways to earn it. I didn't understand what they were exactly, but I thought it all had something to do with not disappointing people. And being useful.

I doubt that my parents intended this. And this doubt helped me to suppress my visceral sense of things. My body knowledge. I learned to ignore how I felt and talked myself into believing that all was well. Unlike most of my friends, I lived with two parents. We had enough to eat. We took vacations. I was going to college. These were the facts.

Then there were my feelings. I felt confused and invisible and unlovable. Because I couldn't reconcile my feelings with the facts, I decided my family was normal but I wasn't—I came out wrong. There was something unacceptable about me and I needed to hide it in order to keep being a part of my family. In the meantime, I had to work harder at becoming acceptable.

After college graduation, I began to sense that I had raised myself. That there were critical pieces of information, instructions, I had never received. And so I looked to peers who seemed to have it together and tried to make my life look like theirs. As an adult, my main concern was blending in.

I felt fake.

And I didn't know how to process feelings, resolve conflict, or tolerate being managed at work. I knew how to isolate and numb myself. These were net effects of the coping strategies I developed as a child. As the strategies became more compulsive and problematic, I picked up new ones. I toggled between them to avoid detection. What I had were addictions. My well-being came down to feeling safe. And my sense of safety was proportional to the amount of control I was able to exert over circumstances and people.

My own body was another story. Here, I had ceded control. Accepting physical contact that I didn't necessarily want was part of fitting in. I was passive, and I didn't understand the rules for sharing touch. Comforting touch and hugs confused me—I soothed myself. As a child I knew that asking for touch meant giving away my last scrap of power. Needing hugs and comfort felt too vulnerable. So I hid my injuries and my upset. Consequently I wasn't comforted. And I was the world's worst hugger. I cut off people's air because I couldn't get the arms right.

When I was twenty-three I was sexually assaulted on a bus, and that sealed the deal. The message from the universe was: my body is not my own. The control I had ceded internally was officially externalized. Everyone could see it. Although I knew that the assault wasn't my fault, I felt ashamed. I began to hide even more of myself and leaned on my unskillful habits to cope.

I stopped dressing nice, unless I had to.

During this period the three feelings I could identify in myself were anger, frustration, and fear. I tried to hide them by being efficient and good. And used my addictions to relieve the pressure. My job became keeping track of what I made up and who knew what. When I was caught in a lie, I told a new one. I couldn't confess. That would mean being wrong, which wasn't safe. Being perfect was safe. Being perfect meant earning the love I craved. Because I still wasn't perfect, I had to work harder.

For me, life was tiny. And it was most definitely without choice. From the time I was small I knew that choice-making could trigger rejection or ridicule. So I let other people choose for me. I seemed easygoing. In fact I was on guard. The tension in my body felt protective. And it was painful. A hard pressure in my solar plexus lit up when I began reaching for what I wanted. It stopped me from choosing in ways that exposed my true self.

My "choice" was whatever freed me from my feelings. The feelings could be good or bad. As time went on, it didn't matter. I didn't want them.

I spent my years in therapy trying to recall facts. Where was the fact that could explain how lost I felt? I listened to family stories, tried to figure out why I couldn't remember events and, more importantly, why they didn't feel relevant to my experience.

Feelings and sensations and impressions can't be quantified. So how can they be true? Objectively my childhood wasn't terrible. This is what I believed. When I was twenty-four a therapist asked me about it. I shared a memory that felt neutral and unremarkable. Wondering, as I spoke, if we would *ever* get to what was *really* bothering me. When I finished, the therapist held silence.

Finally, she said:

"That must have been difficult for a little girl."

Her words surprised me. And they felt correct. I began to consider the possibility that parts of my childhood may have been, empirically speaking, hard. If this were true, perhaps there was something to the free-floating discomfort I carried. And the depression I felt. Perhaps what was *really* bothering me was old pain.

As I write this, I can feel my child self. She is still in there, doing everything in her power to figure out how to feel loved and valuable and seen without understanding that this is what she craves. Every time she fails, she tries again. She is exhausted.

I thought my sense of things was wrong, because none of it matched what I had taught myself to believe. Now I am learning that my sense of things is information, and it's helping me heal. It doesn't matter whose stories it jibes with. And it doesn't matter whether anyone else likes it. My body remembers what's true for me.

My yoga journey began as a bid to manage my anxiety. To burn up feelings and exhaust myself. I was in class almost every day. I was in my forties and only one decade into the habit of taking care of my body. I began when my mom died of a heart attack. She was fifty-seven years old. Inspired by fear, I quit smoking. Then I started exercising. Still I felt anxious. I was hoping yoga would solve that.

Initially it did. Eventually I got injured. And then I got injured again. One day I sustained an injury so bad that I was unable to practice. I received the message—I could not feel my body. And because I couldn't feel my body, I couldn't make choices that were appropriate. The pain of muscle tears and tendonitis was absolutely feelable. But years of numbing had erased the pleasure of being grounded and connected with sensation in a yoga class, or on a hike, or during an awkward hug.

I continued to teach as I healed. As I moved through the familiar shapes I had to make different choices—because I couldn't lift my arm over my head or come into forward bends. This stressed me out. I was there to show people how to do things. And because of my injuries, I was showing them "wrong."

With my high-energy practice on hold, I began exploring yin yoga, and in 2013 I attended a training with Bernie Clark. On a day I will never forget, Bernie asked two participants to come into warrior 2. He adjusted them in the way most of us had been trained to adjust this shape. Then he asked the warriors what they were feeling. One was comfortable. Her hips could do what was required to look perfect in this shape. One was in pain, because her hips wouldn't do what was required to look perfect in this shape— without pain.

I went home feeling moved and unburdened. I didn't have to know how to adjust shapes. I *couldn't* know. In fact it was none of my business. There is no correct version, only yours and mine. My shapes couldn't be wrong because yoga shapes are felt, from the inside out.

When I found Trauma Center Trauma-Sensitive Yoga (TCTSY) I knew I wanted to be of service through yoga in a way that honored what I had learned. On my teacher training application, I wrote that I was done trying to fix people. When I began teaching yoga to survivors, I committed to holding a space for healing. And in holding this space, I've continued my own healing. Working as a TCTSY facilitator has helped me reconnect with the sensation of having a body. To really be in there. Even when it is uncomfortable. Because that is what it takes to facilitate with authenticity.

My primary concern, at first, was to be a good facilitator— perfect, even! However, in order to be present for others, I have to be authentically me. Authentic me will sometimes show up tired or distracted or unable to uphold her vision of perfection. This feels scary. And it gives me pause. If I am committed to meeting clients where they are, why can't I extend that same love to myself?

In a way, I am.

In order to manage my fears while facilitating, I treat the work as an offering—of love and presence and service. I'm learning that I can give these things as though there is an endless supply of goodness inside me. As though *I* am good.

I'm no longer trading love, presence, and service for care. Or attention. Or safety. This seems like self-loving behavior. Actually *feeling* the self-love is still difficult. Accepting that I am lovable, however, is easier.

Facilitating has helped me feel into and appreciate the depth and complexity of my connections to other people. As a child I believed that I could achieve 100 percent self-containment. That I could make myself small enough to avoid pain. I just had to stop needing things. Or people. Or things from people. In many ways I'm still emerging from the habit-energy of trying to live among humans without approaching them. Withdrawing has its own energy. It's quiet, and cold, and people notice. Even if I'm trying to hide, I am readable. We are all experiencing each other. All the time. Invisibly.

So I've never really been alone. And I'm discovering that I don't have to be alone, or in control, in order to feel safe. What's more, I'm learning to tolerate authentic connection with others.

I facilitated TCTSY at a tribal mental health agency for almost two years. At the tribe we didn't talk about trauma. Or use that word. The word itself is a trigger. It conjures up historical trauma, which, for Native People, means genocide. It was coined in the dominant culture. And like the dominant culture, it was imposed. Today it is used, without irony, to describe one outcome of the cultural domination of Native People. So perhaps it's right to let Native People name what that domination feels like or represents, instead of telling them.

I hadn't considered any of this before I was hired. *Trauma* is a word I use. For me, it was baggage-free, and I felt comfortable deploying it to describe bewildering experiences of overwhelm and fear. For other people, it is a roadblock.

A clinician at the tribe gifted me her copy of *Healing the Soul Wound* by Eduardo Duran. In his book, written for counselors working with Native People, Duran writes: "The Native idea of historical trauma involves the understanding that the trauma occurred in the soul or spirit."[1] A wound to the soul. The word *trauma* had always seemed dense enough to encompass the full range of human suffering. As I read these words, and they landed in my body, I realized that it isn't.

Yoga instructor is my baggage-laden phrase. It can conjure up images of youth, fitness, impossible shapes, and the impossibility of certain body types creating those shapes. White women. To call myself a yoga teacher is to provide those who fear yoga for the aforementioned reasons a free pass to reject me out of hand because, although I am no longer youthful, I am Anglo. And I kind of look like a stereotypical yoga teacher.

At the tribe we came up with a new way to describe what I was that did not involve the words *yoga* or *trauma*. I was not the TCTSY person or the yoga lady. I would be the movement specialist. I would offer TCTSY, and modify it, as I got to know the community I was serving.

A few therapists scheduled their adult clients for movement. And the clients wouldn't show up. Each week, at fifteen minutes past appointment time, I would reach out by phone.

"Hello," I would say, "I just wanted to make sure you were alright. We had an appointment today."

"Oh, yes."

"Would you like to reschedule?"

"Yes."

"Is this still a good time?"

"Yes."

"Great," I would say, with a sinking heart, "I'll see you next week."
Next week, they wouldn't show. And I would call again.

My officemates said no-showing was common. They taught me
to send letters inviting people to reengage when they felt ready.
This made me feel better. Maybe it wasn't about me.

I shared space with a group of women who ran programs for
children. We spent a lot of time talking. And learning to trust each
other. Most of them had children. For the first time in a long time,
I started to notice that most women have children. I don't. On
some days, I felt self-conscious about this.

And not everyone wanted to interact with me. I seemed to
offend some people unintentionally. This triggered a survival-
grade dread. For a while I was afraid to go to work. For a while, I
cried in the car every morning as I drove in. I didn't understand
what I was doing wrong. I was pretty sure I just needed to try
harder.

My therapist began to wonder if the job was a good fit for me.
Because I have a long history of leaving jobs at the first sign of
conflict or discomfort, I decided I needed to hang in. And try
harder.

One day an officemate asked me if I'd be willing to teach yoga
at the tribal Head Start summer program. Her confidence in my
potential was all it took to get me to do this thing I never thought I
would consider. Because what did I know about kids?

I have avoided the company of small children for most of my life.

Kids triggered me. They triggered anger and sadness and confusion. I made up a lot of stories about why I didn't want to be around
them. Or have them. But in truth, I was afraid. Afraid of connecting with the sea of body knowledge. My childhood sense of things.
That's where all the pain is.

It's also where my ability to feel joy lives. I figured that out at the Head Start.

There I discovered that my fear of children was literally visceral. They ignited a body sense of the powerlessness and despair I felt as a child. I could see how much love and attention and nurturing children need to thrive. On days when I felt secure and sane, I was able to picture myself small, and entirely dependent on my care-givers. I could see how hard I had worked to care for myself. And I started to feel some self-compassion.

Tracking my sensations and staying with my body while facilitating showed me that I can stay present in the face of one of my oldest triggers. I was also learning to feel safe in authenticity. The kids were my teachers. They showed me something I had forgotten—children are willing to be wild and curious and uninhibited and vulnerable. Until they learn it's not a good idea.

I could not remember feeling wild and curious and uninhibited way down in my viscera. However, I would be teaching yoga to very large classes of tiny people who terrified me—so I would be practic-ing vulnerability along with the kids.

My route at the Head Start led me through classrooms of kids aged three through six. I created short sequences with a simple story and shapes that could be plants or animals that had positive or neutral associations for tribal members. Each sequence was tailored to the age group, and each week I brought a song or a chant we would sing together—because I read that small children like to sing. I am not a singer. But I committed to singing. And to making animal sounds, if that seemed necessary.

My singing debut was with the three-year-olds and their teach-ers. I sat in the circle, awash in sweat, mumbling the first verse of my chant, slowly, introducing the arm movements I invented behind the closed doors of my office.

A little sun,

A little shower,

A little while and then . . . a flower.

Arms behind my head, still a sunflower, I paused to look around the circle. I saw twenty-five confused faces. A room packed with three-year-olds had fallen silent.

The two teachers waited, arms behind their heads, as though it were the most natural thing in the world to be a sunflower.

Look at me! I thought. *Am I someone who sings and does make believe? I can't do it!* I wanted to drop through the floor.

Then one of the teachers, in that magical way that preschool teachers do, picked up the chant and sang as though they had composed it. Soon there were twenty-five chanting sunflowers. Together we pretended to be the sun and the rain and sprouting seeds.

As I picked up my gear and walked toward the door, I felt as though I could do anything. Only four more classrooms to go.

By the end of the summer, I was a singer. The six-year-olds were requesting "Twinkle, Twinkle, Little Star" and singing it twice—once in English and again in their tribal language. And they wanted to teach me the version I didn't know.

I ended each class with a chime and created an opportunity for the kids to feel their breath moving. I placed my hands on my abdomen and invited the children to do the same. I shared that when I felt upset or angry, I might sit just like they we were sitting and see if I could notice my abdomen moving. And I told them that sometimes, after a while, the upset or the anger passed.

Then I invited the chime. We listened in silence until the sound was no longer audible. For the first few weeks the novelty of a near-silent classroom tempted a number of kids to exercise their outdoor voices inside. But soon the chime sang in silence. Some kids began listening with their eyes closed, so they could focus on the final tones. One by one, they raised their hands when they could no longer hear the chime.

I used the word *invite* to describe the moment when the mallet met the chime. More than one child asked me why I didn't say "hit." "The chime is a friend," I said. "I like to invite my friends to sing with me." It was an opportunity to talk about asking rather than taking, gentleness as opposed to force. Invitation versus command. The chime is our friend and we're asking it to sing for us. The chime would not be forced to sing.

And preschoolers would not be forced to be trees or frogs.

This was what I wanted.

However, the kids were often forced to be trees and frogs. At the beginning of my second summer I met with the teachers and asked that they not rearrange the limbs of children who weren't doing exactly what I was doing. And I shared my reasoning—there are infinite ways to be a flower.

Adults, with words and touch, spend a lot of time deciding what kids should be doing with their bodies. When kids practice authentic choice through movement, they get to have a felt experience of being in charge of their own bodies. This can be especially powerful for kids living with unstable caregivers. For them the survival-level project is tracking the environment and the adults who populate it. Eventually they stop noticing what is happening inside themselves. They sacrifice their sense of self and their agency in order to keep safe. When a child decides where to put their arms and how deeply to bend, they are turning inward for guidance. Not toward the adults in the room. They are expressing self-responsibility. They are in control of what happens to them. And all of this starts from noticing how their body wants to make a flower.

Some kids came to Head Start with behavioral coaches. Children with delays received hands-on attention. These were special cases. But it seemed clear to me that just because a child was not doing what I was doing didn't mean they weren't participating. There was some watching. Some waiting. Some curiosity. And shyness. I wanted all of those kids to be in charge of their own limbs. To be free to join when they were ready and inspired.

I was asking a lot of these teachers who were managing overfull classrooms and a fair number of children with "heart loss, thought loss," or behavioral challenges.

And I related to the teachers who wanted to run a tight ship. That was me.

I spent ten years teaching in secondary and adult education. My strategy for getting through each day boiled down to controlling my students. During the year I taught high school full time, I was not able to secure enough control over my students to feel safe. I was afraid of being challenged, afraid of being inadequate, afraid of being wrong. I abandoned myself. Instead I focused on them. I clamped down. At the time, I didn't know how to do better. At the time, I had no idea that the control I was so keen to exercise was eroding my ability to connect. I was in my own silo. I wasn't available to my students.

Facilitating has shown me that I don't have to control people in order to feel safe around them. Choosing what is right for me, while observing others make their own choices, reinforces this over and over again. What I observe is that I'm usually okay, no matter what other people are doing.

Each shape in TCTSY is an opportunity to practice choice-making. As I facilitate, I flag options for choice. For example, in a given shape, one choice might be practicing with your arms on your hips. A second choice might be stretching your arms to the side. As I move, I am making my own decisions about where to put my arms. In a class of ten, I might look up and see ten different versions of the shape I offered. I might see ten different shapes. Or motion. Or someone following along with me. My job is to create space for all of it.

It's a humbling practice for day-to-day living to watch someone choose what they want and then deal with my feelings about it. I always have feelings about it. Why? Does it affect my safety? No. Sometimes it can feel like it does.

Everyone's choices are fluid and evolving. In fact we are one big system in flux. I can't have certainty. I can only change along with everyone else.

I'm slowly releasing my expectation that I can feel secure by keeping the world around me static. Checking in with my body, responding to it authentically, is a built-in safety valve that helps me keep my eyes on me. So even when I'm nervous, I'm present. If something comes up that needs my attention, I flex, instead of snapping in two. Or freezing.

The six-year-olds were seated, hands on their abdomens, listening to the chime. It was the last class of my first summer at Head Start. I was feeling relieved, sad, excited. Worried. I still had very little to do at the tribe.

As the sound faded, one child raised their hand—to show me that they couldn't hear the chime. That was what I thought.

Then, they started talking.

"I was at the store with my mom last week and she was really mad . . ."

An unscripted moment. My first impulse, residue from classroom teaching, was *shut it down*. Because was this going to be a story that ended badly? Instead I focused on my abdomen moving.

". . . *really* mad . . ."

I looked at the teachers. They seemed content to let the moment unfold. I focused on my abdomen, moving.

". . . so I said, 'Sometimes, when I'm upset, I put my hand on my belly, and try to feel my breath. And it helps me feel better.'"

The words I said at the end of each class.

I had felt awkward saying these words. Just as awkward as I felt singing and making animal sounds and being silly. I was practicing new skills, trying things out with an audience. All of this brought up shame.

The kids didn't roll their eyes or laugh when I leapt like a frog or roared like a lion. They leapt and roared. When I reached for the chime at the end of class, they put their hands on their bellies. They waited for the tone. They trusted me enough to try new things. And one of them took something new out into the world and shared it with someone else.

It was completely unexpected.

I decided to try and spend more time at the Head Start.

The next summer, I convinced the Head Start administrators to allow me to work one-on-one with some of the children. Although the teachers wanted to send me the kids with "heart loss, thought loss," I encouraged them to consider the kids who seemed withdrawn, afraid, or shy. Which can also be signs of distress.

My inaugural client was a four-year-old. I invited them into an office that had been stripped of every potentially distracting item. I asked whether they'd like the door open or closed. Whether they'd like a pink or purple mat. I had four cards ready. The child chose one. I looked at the card, and I saw an intense back bend:

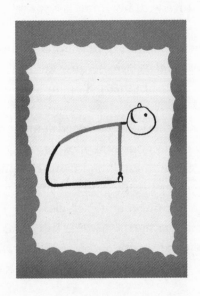

In an instant, I remembered how hard I worked to get into and out of this shape "correctly." Recalled the moment I gave up performing the shape "fully"—to protect my neck. The disappointment I felt with my "incomplete" version. *Could I do this shape without warming up?* I wondered.

Then I saw the child—on their belly.

I checked the card. And saw: And . . . the child saw:

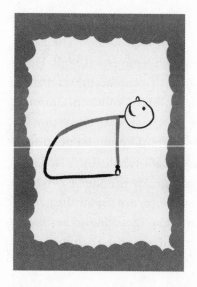 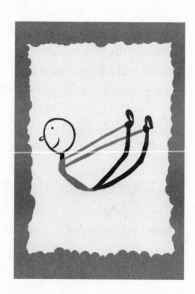

They read the card upside-down. For them, there was no top or bottom. No right way or wrong way. The card was readable from all sides, awash in possibilities that I had never noticed. Because I was trained—to see the kneeling backbend.

We tried out all of the options, which set off a giggle avalanche. This was not the final child to rotate a card through its full 360 degrees of possibility.

Adults are charged with keeping kids safe and teaching them pretty much everything they need to know to thrive. This involves creating a limited, age-appropriate menu of options for them. Kids have fewer choices. And yet they can see more possibility in a shape than I do—as long as I don't snatch the card out of their hand and say, "No, honey, it goes like this."

At the Head Start I learned how easily I can impose my own fears and limitations on the imagination and curiosity of a young person. And at the home for tribal youth, I discovered that my emotions are, in fact, tangible. I communicate them on an energetic level, without saying a word.

My longest assignment at the tribe was facilitating in a house for tribal youths who had been removed from their homes. The house usually had six boys in residence, and the turnover was high. Holding a group movement class was what made sense to my managers, so I tried that. Then I had grounds to lobby for my preference: one-on-one sessions.

I began using yoga cards and the ten-minute model developed by David Emerson. The level of participation still fluctuated, but individual decisions about how to engage, or whether to engage, occurred in the semi-privacy of the day room, not under the gaze of fellow residents and the adults on duty. Each session was an opportunity to disengage from the house and spend one-on-one time with an adult who would not be asking them to talk or problem-solve or do.

Working with the youths was one of the most deeply gratifying things I have ever done. I prided myself on being fully present for them week after week. My essential role was to show up on time, to call when I couldn't be there, and to be the same Kirsten each time I walked through the door. In other words, my job was to be predictable and reliable and safe. Whether the youths chose to participate or not, no matter how noisy it was, I was calm and centered.

Until one day.

Less than half an hour before I was scheduled to work, I received very upsetting news. I had time to sit by myself, to breathe, to get out of my head and into my body. I thought I took care of it. And then I went to work. From the beginning, something felt off. Each youth chose fewer shapes than was usual for them and spent less time with me. No one asked me about my day. No one wanted to chat. There was no eye contact.

I thought the house dynamic was off. I wondered whether something had happened right before I walked in—until my biggest fan came to choose cards. This was the youth who always wanted to participate, the only youth who shared what they felt in their body as they moved. They came in, practiced, and left.

The common denominator was me. As I walked to my car, I began to unravel. I had been burning up energy just to stay calm. I had facilitated each card and offered interoceptive cues based on what I felt in my own body. The same as always. Or so I thought. The youths sensed a shift in the quality of my presence. And they knew what I was feeling even before I did—I was angry.

They were giving me room. I felt terrible.

Because I remember what it was like to sense anger rolling off adults, knowing I had to fix it or get out of the way. Knowing I had to choose correctly. Mostly I got out of the way. I hid in stories, in trees, in closets, at my friends' houses. Mostly I hid who I was and put my false self forward. It became my default.

The youths, all of whom had lived through terrible things and had trained themselves to notice shifts and changes in people, were on to me.

I have only had this one experience of facilitating-while-angry. In the wake of it, I realized something important. On all the other weeks, weeks when I had arrived at the house filled with joy and gratitude for this job, excited to see the youths, I had been my authentic self. It was becoming habitual and unconscious. Even better, I was learning that being that person could feel safe and good.

The day I told the youths that I would not be working with them any longer was the hardest day. Harder than all the days I cried on the drive to work. And it was one of the best days, because I knew that our time together had mattered to them. They let me *see* that it mattered to them, because I had let them see *me*.

When I'm offering choice in a session, I'm admitting that I don't know what you need, because I am not you.

And I'm engaging with myself so that I can offer authentic cues. I ground, and I manage myself.

I'm available to you, but I'm not available to manage you or save you.

Providing authentic choice is the difference between rescuing and offering help.

I keep myself honest by staying in my own body and noticing what is coming up as I facilitate. Usually fear is what is coming up. Fear of getting it wrong.

I can't get this wrong. As long as I keep my focus on my practice, there is room for you to have yours.

When I first began with yoga, there were teachers I felt safe with and teachers I avoided. I couldn't explain my preferences in a way that would satisfy anyone else—but I sensed what I needed. Ultimately, as a non-tribal person working for an Indian tribe, I realized that the most qualified facilitator is not necessarily the one with the certification; it's the person clients feel safest with. And that might be another tribal member.

Choosing to work with me, just like choosing one shape over another, is a choice. And we're all in charge of making our own. It wasn't a matter of selling myself or TCTSY more effectively. I didn't need to try harder. Once I saw this clearly, I stopped pushing. I was learning the difference between forcing and allowing.

Understanding the source of my own pain was paradigm-altering. And it doesn't qualify me to understand or resolve the suffering of others. As the movement specialist I had expertise in a certain area— but I was not an expert on anyone's pain but mine.

By the time I was hired by the tribe, I had stopped minimizing my wounds by comparing myself to others. I could accept that what I felt was real and that it had prevented me from growing in a lot of fundamental ways.

Healing, in part, meant learning to see my choices. Recognizing that I'm a grown-up and have options that the child-me didn't have. For years I couldn't see this.

Many of the tribal members I worked with or facilitated for were carrying the imprints of adverse childhood experiences in their bodies. And, unlike me, they are also living in a larger system that perpetuates their pain in myriad ways.

I can identify with adverse childhood experiences. With the experience of being a woman in this culture. But I am not a woman of color. I haven't endured the slow drip of race-based microaggression. And I don't know what it's like to try to heal in a country that, not so long ago, tried to eliminate my forbearers. I don't carry the body memory of genocide.

As someone who, half a century on, is still trying to figure out how to love herself, this realization can feel threatening. I grew up believing in the economy of deprivation—if there is enough for you there is, by default, nothing left for me. There is not enough love or support, security or compassion, to go around. There are winners and losers. Sadly this is still one of the dominant narratives of my culture.

And I have a choice. I can choose to view life as cooperative, not competitive.

I know that as I recognize the suffering of others—even if I can't relate, even if it seems worse than my own—I still get to acknowledge and release my own stuff.

There is room for everyone's pain. There is enough compassion to go around.

All of us get to heal.

In my body there is lingering fear that this isn't true—for me. Facilitating has shown me that it *is* true. The practice itself is a visceral experience of making space for everyone, including myself. Of interacting with others and maintaining an open heart.

We offer each other help and support by moving our individual stories in community, each of us attending to our own bodies. Taking care of ourselves first. This is diametrically opposed to what I learned to do as a child.

We're not each of us trying to heal alone. Instead we are creating a container that can hold and honor each individual experience of suffering. Everyone's history is an essential and valued part
of a new whole that we shape together.

Every time I facilitate I touch into the sense that I am co-creating
with people I can't see or imagine. Nothing I do occurs in a vacuum.
My actions impact you; your actions impact me. When I take care
of my pain, I help you through yours. No matter how alone I feel,
there you are. And you. And you. And we're all in this together.
And it's always been this way.

Moving in Authentic Relationship

Beyond Immigration to Healing and Connection

Gwen Soffer

A KEY COMPONENT TO FACILITATING a yoga class is the spoken word—commanding students to create precise shapes with their bodies, instructing micro-corrections of arms, legs, hips, muscles, joints, and even directing how someone is breathing. In Western classes there is focus on doing the pose "correctly," and the teacher is given complete control as the expert of the practice. The expectation is that the teacher will be wise, commanding, and inspirational and will provide a complete mind-body experience in sixty to ninety minutes. Under this pressure to prove myself as valid and worthy of my title as yoga teacher, I had spent years crafting my language for my public studio classes. Initially my instruction was clumsy and overacted, trying too much to sound like what I had been taught a yoga teacher should sound like—knowledgeable and always in control. Ironically, once I gained more experience and confidence, I realized that the more I tried to fit the mold of what was expected of a good teacher, the less it was true. Only when I learned to show up as myself—humble, imperfect, and authentically experiencing the present moment just like my students were—and not as the all-knowing figure that I thought was expected of me, did I become a good teacher.

I can remember exactly when this happened for me. For the first time, I went into class without a script, without a plan, and led the class trusting that I knew what to say next. More importantly, instead of following a preconceived plan, I stayed in tune with what was happening with the participants in the class, assessing their energy levels, their emotional states, their unspoken needs in each moment. I was no longer reciting words but rather letting them flow in response to what was happening right in front of me. At the end of the class I realized that I was much more at ease than usual. My body was not tense, and my thoughts were not heavy. Instead of spending energy formulating what I was going to say because I thought it was expected, I was actually being myself. What I felt was relief—the relief that comes when you let your guard down, and you allow other people to see you. In a sense I felt as if I too had participated in the yoga class and was reaping the benefit of being in the present moment.

After so many years of trying to sound like an expert, I realized that authenticity, not command, is at the heart of being a yoga teacher. To be in relationship with your students you have to work to let go of the need for others to accept you as the expert. This allows you to be seen, and that builds trust, which is the foundation of a shared authentic experience. In many traditional Western yoga classes, the teacher is positioned to be the giver of knowledge and wisdom, and the student the unquestioning receiver of the teacher's expertise—a remnant of historical guru culture. Underneath this dynamic is an imbalance of power, as the teacher is rarely vulnerable and the student always is. What I had experienced during that pivotal class was me expressing vulnerability, not trying to prove anything, but rather sharing a piece of myself that was not rehearsed. I was being, not posturing. I was speaking without pretense, not pontificating. I was standing with my students, not over them. I can be introverted, so letting down the expert mask I was hiding behind was intimidating at first, but once I felt the relief of not needing or even wanting to be perfect, there was no turning back. The gap between the persona I had created as a teacher and who I am as a person had closed. I could show up to class ready to have a shared authentic experience with my students instead of performing to a crowd. These experiences happen when we allow others to see that we do not have all the answers and that we are navigating the present moment with the same uncertainty as our students.

I serve as the wellness coordinator at the Nationalities Service Center (NSC), where we work with clients from over 110 countries. Our clients speak multiple languages and have varied religions, cultural norms, and practices. My role is to coordinate onsite clinical and holistic services, including Wellness Wednesday when we offer clients free trauma-sensitive yoga, acupuncture, and massage as well as other therapeutic services. Although I had taught yoga for over fifteen years, there were some unique and practical considerations when I first started the group. My current yoga group, for example, consists of clients from Democratic Republic of the Congo (DRC), Rwanda, Iran, Iraq, Afghanistan, Syria, Pakistan, Algeria, Bhutan, Haiti, Mexico, and Guatemala. Some are newer to the country and speak very little English, and others have been in the US for a few years but have limited English. Some have refugee and asylum status, and others are working through long and complicated legal asylum cases.

The commonality among all is the level of complex trauma and extreme loss they have experienced amid the stress of relocating into a new country far from their home. The layers of trauma are deep. There are personal experiences of violence, sexual assault, torture, witnessing the same of their loved ones, and loss of family, home, livelihood, and all that is familiar. Then there is the larger collective trauma felt by whole communities—exposure to war and violence in home countries and the loss of culture, country, customs, and connection, in addition to experiences of discrimination, xenophobia, and racism that happens during displacement and relocation in another country. The original trauma that leads people to flee their home is compounded by the extreme traumatic stress of resettling in an unfamiliar place, often into financial insecurity, where they have to simultaneously learn the language, gain employment, navigate complicated social, medical, and legal systems, and rebuild their lives—usually without appropriate mental health support or opportunities for healing. The specifics of their lives vary, but the group participants understand their shared experience of loss, trauma, relocation, and isolation.

> I find Wellness Wednesday relaxing. It is nice to talk to new people and is stress reducing. Also the employees help me a lot. I enjoy all of the activities. I find it nice to be around people instead of being alone. I enjoy meeting with the group and to have the opportunity to meet with new people from different countries. Wellness Wednesday does reduce my stress amidst living in a new country.   —Participant from Pakistan

When I walked into my first yoga session at NSC, I had decided that the best way to be trauma sensitive was to not have a rigid expectation of how the session would go or what it would look like, but instead to be truly in the present moment. It meant going in with my training and knowledge of trauma but not letting it be the epicenter of the group experience.

I do not know the specific stories of the people who attend the yoga group, but I know that the level of trauma they have experienced is profound, so I use TCTSY trauma-sensitive protocols. To build trust and create safety for the group, I need to show gentle, non-coercive understanding and kindness. I also know I need to allow the dynamic of the group to guide us forward instead of forcing my conception of what the group would be. This means being aware of any power dynamic that may mimic past coercive experiences and ensuring that people have choice and control in the practice. This means being aware of the physical, emotional, psychological, and human-rights violations that people may have experienced, including torture, assault, and deprivation, and how this can manifest in their experience of their own body. This means being aware of people's complex need to protect themselves yet also connect with others, and how trauma can profoundly affect trust within relationships. It also means understanding how trauma can affect every aspect of people's lives while also being aware of cultural differences that could lead to insult, offense, or mistrust. I must be willing to embrace the unknown and allow the group to evolve at its own pace in order to ensure the practice is serving them and not me.

All the years I had spent perfecting my "yoga voice" would not serve me now as I entered into a circle of survivors where I could not rely on my language to convey meaning, but rather I had to walk softly in order to gain their trust. Not only did I not speak the languages represented in the room, but my asserting power, as is inherent in the commanding voice we are taught in our yoga teacher trainings, would be both harmful and alienating. I led the women through a gentle chair yoga sequence, speaking in simple sentences and moving through the forms with them. It was liberating to break the forms down to the basics instead of describing in detail how each movement was "supposed" to be performed, as would be common in a public yoga class, and we were free to experience the movements in our own way.

In the time that I have been offering yoga at NSC, I have seen how prevalent somatic expression of trauma is among clients—headaches, back pain, stomachaches, muscle soreness. It is important to understand that these pains can be the result of emotional and psychological trauma as well as physical trauma, because our clients' trauma histories are multileveled. The women in the group are expressive about what they are feeling, saying "ah!" when stretching or "oh!" if something is uncomfortable. They frequently point to the place where they are feeling pain, and I offer a gentle reminder to take it slow. This surprised me at first because the focus of trauma theories is often on the dissociation from body sensation that is very common in trauma survivors. The women in the group, however, are very vocal about what they are feeling and can clearly communicate these sensations even without the English words.

In addition to verbal expression of physical sensation, there is a lot of laughing during the practice. Even though we can't always rely on our words to express ourselves in the group, there is a lot of humor. Like the time we were doing a forward fold, and I realized that I had been walking around all day with my boots unzipped. As we were folded forward, I zipped up my boots, and the women were so amused they began to laugh. Or the times when the older Iraqi woman in the group makes a joke in Arabic, and even though many of us are not sure what she said, her intent of humor is clear, and we all laugh with her. Or when we have our arms reaching to the center of the circle during a yoga pose, and I say, "Say hi to your neighbor," and we all begin to wave and say hello to the person across from us. There are plenty of these beautiful, humorous moments, and we embrace them as part of our connection and our healing. In a public yoga class this would be considered a disruption, but here it is a full expression of freedom, authenticity, and experiencing your body in the present moment.

We have very limited space, so we run the group in a multifunctional classroom where there are lots of tables and chairs. In the early days, I would have to arrive twenty minutes before the start time to set up the room, but now the women in the group set it up on their own, patiently waiting until I arrive. The participants take pride and ownership of the space, as well as gratification in contributing to the group, by helping to set up and break down the room. This is particularly poignant given that they have lost their own homes and have experienced such immense lack of control of their environment in the past. They are enthusiastic to have the group and want to be part of its creation.

Each Wednesday is a bit different, but a core group is there each week: eight women from Pakistan, Iran, Iraq, DRC, Rwanda, Algeria, Haiti, and Mexico. They greet each other with big smiles and warm hugs, speaking in limited English and mixing in their native languages. I had made the decision early on not to use interpretation, and now I barely notice the language difference as we all help each other understand. Not only is interpretation very costly—and we have so many languages represented in the group that it would be impractical—but it also creates further separation when you are speaking through a third person. With no interpretation, we are all on the same level as we find our way through multiple languages, expert in our own, but not in another. One participant says that we don't need interpretation because "we speak the language of the heart, and smiles are the same in all languages." Living in a country where you are not fluent in the language is very stressful and often makes people feel insecure and separated. Communicating without interpretation allows us to work it out together—another shared authentic experience. It also provides reinforcement of the participants' growing English skills. There is a part of the chair sequence when we lift one leg and make movements with our ankles and feet. One of the participants from Mexico always says out loud, "Point and flex," as she has proudly learned these words from hearing me say them so many times. Now it has become a group joke, and when we get to that movement, everyone says loudly, "Point and flex," and we all chuckle.

Along with the joy that is expressed in the group is unconditional support. Often someone will come to the group struggling with something—the loss of a loved one back home, an illness of a family member, financial difficulties, an overwhelming legal matter. Within moments the members become aware of the distressed person and circle around to comfort her with soothing words or gentle hugs. I have noticed that the women are very comfortable with physical touch. Recently a woman was crying because of a legal matter that was affecting her family and causing her great worry. Another woman, who was from a completely different culture, came over and sweetly took the woman's face in her hands and gave her a kiss on the check. I watched the interaction, wondering how the crying woman would react because they had not known each other long. In that moment she leaned in and rested her head on the other woman's shoulder. There was no hesitation from either woman, just a spontaneous expression of connection and humanity. I can always tell when I walk into the room and the woman are circled around that they have joined together to support someone in need.

Whenever I see people working and exercising during these . . . services, it helps me not think about a lot of stress. I enjoy the group because I am able to chat and learn among different people. My husband works a lot, so there is a lot of burden on him to take care of the family. I think about this a lot. Each time has gotten worse. When I come here and meet new people. I feel the group is consoling and helps me stop thinking.
                                                    —Participant from Rwanda

This type of support and shared experience is common in the group. Periodically one of the women brings a child, who sits in the center of the circle and plays. All of the women look after the child in a way that conveys that communal care is a cultural norm and is no different in the yoga room. Nobody is annoyed and everyone sees it as quite normal. The women all care for the children, handing them toys, offering them a piece of fruit, helping them up onto chairs, and gently redirecting them when they run around. By the end of the class, the child is going up to anyone in the group to show them something they found, to smile, or to simply lean on their lap. It is a heartwarming display of a collectivist approach to community that is so different from the more typical individualist approach in the US. There is no mom-shaming or expectation that the mom will make the child be quiet. The child becomes part of the group for the day. One time we were sitting in our ending meditation, and a young Syrian boy was singing the ABCs in the background. It was the perfect melody to accompany the class, and it enhanced the experience for all of us.

Sometimes phones go off, someone arrives late, or there is a noise in the hallway. In a yoga studio these would be considered unacceptable and worthy of reprimand, but this does not bother us, and we continue to go through the gentle movements regardless of the distractions that may arise. There is an acceptance of life happening around us during the yoga class, and designing a pristine environment is not what creates peace for the group. The women in the group have experienced unimaginable chaos that turned their lives upside down, and the disarray of everyday moments like these is not enough to disrupt the experience. It is a reminder that these moments of peace are in front of us all the time, even in the midst of commotion, and we don't need to create the perfect environment in order to experience them.

I take yoga class every time . . . I like yoga. I came when I have a problem with my knee and back. The pain has gone down after doing yoga. It also helps with stress . . . I have many papers to fill, and they make me so busy I can't think. But yoga, I really like it. I came from Africa, and I think too much. Yoga helps me wind down. I can talk to people. I feel American. I see my life. I really appreciate it. You meet your friends, you talk, and you do exercise. I enjoy. It changed my life. Big change.

—Lolie, Democratic Republic of the Congo

Lolie is a mother of three who came to the US with refugee status from DRC. Lolie's case manager had suggested that she try yoga, so she came to the Wednesday group. During her first class she was quiet and did not engage with me much. As we began the session, she moved tentatively through the sequence. The next week she came back and greeted me with a smile. She continued to come back every week thereafter, and now when I see her she gives me a big "Hello!" Even when I see her in the hallway as she waits for her appointment with her case manager, she stops me, lifts her arms to the sky and says, "Yoga today?" My favorite memory with Lolie is one day when she came to NSC not knowing that we had cancelled yoga because of expected bad weather. She saw me walking down the hallway and asked, "Yoga today?" I told her that even though the group would not be there that day, we could do a session if she liked. She smiled and agreed, and we found an available room. We moved through the sequence together, and the whole time she had a gentle smile and so did I. As we sat in our ending meditation, I realized that I had not gotten refreshments as I usually do because the class had technically been cancelled. When we finished, I looked in my bag and there were two clementine oranges left over from the previous week. I pulled them out, and we sat facing each other, eating our clementine in silence—a true shared authentic experience, no words needed.

Murielle, a client from Ivory Coast, was originally referred to clinical therapy, but she did not want to continue because she did "not want to talk about the past because it made it worse." She had come to the yoga group several times, and when her case manager asked if she might want to try a private yoga session with me, she agreed. She said that she wanted to come because "she feels good around the teacher." I realized then just how important the connection is between service providers and clients, and that Murielle was only willing to try private yoga sessions because she trusted me. This trust is critical especially with people who have experienced abuse and violation to the extent that Murielle had. It is not enough to show up with expertise; we need to also show up as a relatable person who is safe, supportive, consistent, and kind. She needed to feel safe in order to be vulnerable, and being with the right person was significant to her. Since then, I meet with her weekly for private sessions, and other than our initial greeting at the beginning, we do not speak much. It is enough to be together, gently moving through the forms and breathing together.

Murielle demonstrates many physical symptoms, and when I go to the waiting room to bring her back to the yoga room, she has difficulty standing up and appears to be in pain with each step, but she always gives me a big smile when I greet her. We begin the yoga session sitting in a chair facing each other, and with that first deep breath together, her body completely changes. She closes her eyes, sits up tall, her breath slows, and she has a subtle smile. As we begin the forms, she moves her arms with intention and focus, and at the end of the practice, as we sit quietly and breathe, her body is calm, her energy is at ease, and she seems completely at peace, graceful and free.

The biggest lesson I have learned facilitating yoga sessions at NSC is that moments of peace cannot be created through planning and emphasis on structure. Instead, acceptance of the aftermath of trauma and a commitment to the nurturing of authentic human connection are what allow for healing. These shared authentic experiences only happen when we are humble, open, and vulnerable. If we enter a room with the belief that we know more or have more expertise and experience, we perpetuate separation, and we lose the valuable opportunity to learn from the experiences of others. I am extremely grateful to be part of this circle of women and to learn from their generosity, strength, and kindness and their willingness to find healing with each other in the everyday moment.

> Yoga is good exercise for my body and mind. I feel very alive.
> —Participant from Algeria

Paralleled Agency

Inside the Safe Relationship

Emily Lapolice

MIRIAM ACHED WITH A HEAVINESS that pulsed through her bones. With limbs that felt like lead, she found herself hostage in her own body, the fatigue forcing conditions of captivity. Perhaps only making it out of bed for a few hours a day was not at all an uncommon experience. Any longer than that, though offering an enticing glimpse of what her "old life" used to feel like, would carry consequences. She may, for example, be laid up for days, unable to get out of bed any longer than it takes to use the facilities, reach for a half-eaten protein bar on the bedside table, and return to bed. Functions of basic survival.

Myalgic encephalomyelitis (ME), commonly known as chronic fatigue syndrome (CFS), is a debilitating and complex illness affecting up to 2.5 million Americans, many of whom remain undiagnosed and suffer in a bewildering silence.[1] As people who have ME/CFS often appear physically "well," experiencing a kaleidoscope of symptoms that many health-care professionals misunderstand or may not take seriously, many refer to the disease as an "invisible illness." Miriam is also a breast cancer survivor and has spoken many times about the vast difference between her battle with cancer and her daily fight for survival with ME/CFS. She references the wide range of support she felt during her cancer treatment, from pink ribbons to the "casseroles of chemotherapy," as she called them, that are starkly absent in the relentless reality that is now her life. Those who suffer from ME/CFS experience overwhelming fatigue that is not improved by rest and made worse by *any* amount of activity—physical or mental. Miriam has spoken of a distinct kind of exhaustion she experiences on a daily basis from having to "pay such close attention to everything," feeling the effects of this exertion on a cellular level.

During our work together, Miriam has shared many in-depth and poignant glimpses into what living with a chronic illness like this looks and feels like. One such example is when she speaks about "efforting" and the "conversion energy" it takes to perform simple basic tasks. She describes *conversion energy* as the laborious energy or effort it takes to convert internalized step-by-step processes—which are, for most people, often done automatically—toward an effective action-based skill or task (motor planning, for example). Thinking through the steps of what items she may need at a grocery store to prepare a meal, not to mention how to get to the grocery store and by which mode of transportation (she primarily relies on car services despite the financial burden, as they remain the only reliable way to get herself anywhere), can be paralyzing for Miriam or evoke intense panic attacks. She describes an "avalanche" quality to her distressing emotions of grief, anxiety, and self-loathing, ensuing deep feelings of helplessness and hopelessness.

Despite once being a successful film producer often specifically sought out for her innate ability to multitask and hold ideas and concepts with such a skilled perspective, envisioning the end result long before its arrival, Miriam has lost the ability to engage with life in this way any longer. Since any amount of "tasking" is susceptible to so many variables and triggers, both physical and psychological, completing tasks is nearly impossible. The energy she expends on every detail of her life (basic decision-making, physical movement and coordination, activities of daily living, the dynamics of relational interactions) feels constant and relentless—a continual cycle of depletion with very little opportunity for restoration or recovery. Award-winning author Laura Hillenbrand suffers from the disease and describes the exhaustion as being "so profound it's a struggle to breathe, a struggle to just lie there; it takes every effort just to stay alive. This can go on for months or years . . . You have to be so careful with every little bit of energy. You just don't know where your line is."[2] Miriam references this "line" creating such stark opposition in her life, because her mood, energy, and overall functioning can fluctuate from extreme agitation/activation to a near-catatonic state. An illness of this kind has conditions, implications, and impacts on the physical and psychological body that are complexly traumatic in nature. It is isolating, uncomfortable, filled with shame, and devoid of purpose. But what intensifies this landscape even more for Miriam is that her experience of ME/CFS is not the only traumatic aspect of her life. Severe chronic illness makes recovery from the pileup of prior losses and trauma extremely difficult. Experts in the ME/CFS field now universally agree that people who have this illness can no longer normally process stress. It negatively affects nearly every system in the body—immune, endocrine, the brain and nervous system, for starters. Added stress is extremely harmful, and they warn of possible permanent damage to neurocognitive and metabolic energy functioning.[3] But Miriam's day-to-day life is inherently stressful.

She has endured sustained trauma and assault on her body, mind, and psyche multiple times over the course of her life. What distinguishes complex trauma from post-traumatic stress disorder (most often a response to a single-episode traumatic event) is the chronicity and repetitive nature of trauma, usually occurring within the context of relationships. Miriam was a child of intergenerational trauma; her father, a Jewish refugee during the Holocaust, was authoritarian, shaming, and abusive; her mother, emotionally vacant and unattuned. She was also a victim of sexual assault as a young adult and endured a traumatic birth experience during the delivery of her only son. Her husband's untreated addiction ultimately contributed to the demise of their relationship, his homelessness, and his gruesome and untimely death. A death that happened shortly after Miriam lost her closest friend to cancer—the same cancer she had only just recently fought and survived herself. The man she met and fell in love with after her divorce left her after nearly a decade together, at one of the most challenging times of her illness. This triggered intense abandonment anxiety and may have been part of the impetus for Miriam to seek treatment with me. Excerpts from her initial inquiry email reveal the longevity, chronicity, and severity of the layers of trauma she has experienced:

I am looking for a clinician and yoga practitioner to work with around the stress and isolation of chronic illness, a series of multiple traumatic losses, complicated grief, and emotion and somatic regulation. I struggle with sleep disturbance, ME/CFS, post cancer treatment cognitive deficits, depression and anxiety. I am unemployed after decades of meaningful work in film. I have a therapist who is mostly engaged in supportive therapy and a psychopharmacologist who has me on quite a lot of psychotropic medication, but I am stuck: In grief, sadness and fear.

My entire personality has been altered. I am extremely easily overwhelmed. Sensory and perceptually overloaded. Highly emotionally reactive, impulsive, and cognitively challenged. My judgement is poor. I feel awash in my emotions. Never at peace. And to the detriment of my relationships: irritate easily, reactive and panicky. Lost in a perpetual state of disorganization . . . and replaying past losses and trauma, unable to remain in the present or fully mourn and move on from the significant losses I have suffered.

It is impossible to make sense of my symptoms. Physical, neurological, cognitive, psychological, or medication related? I know this. I feel stuck in an uncomfortable limbic state from which I do not seem to be able to ground myself.

I have always been a physical person. I have lost that person, almost entirely. Over the course of the last decade, post cancer and with the sometimes debilitating exhaustion of ME/CFS—I also have lost touch with my body. I strongly believe the place to begin "recovery" for me is in the body. . . .

When I received this email, I was already in awe of the woman behind the computer screen: her intelligence and astute self-awareness, despite feeling such an utter and profound loss of self; her vulnerability, courage, and authenticity; and the multilayered fabric of her unique lived experience. Miriam had heard of Trauma Center Trauma-Sensitive Yoga (TCTSY) when she sought me out as her therapist, but she knew little more than it being a body-based treatment designed for complex trauma. Never intended to take the place of psychotherapy, TCTSY can be used as an adjunctive modality to psychotherapy or, in our case, a combined approach of utilizing TCTSY within the psychotherapy relationship. Miriam had been in psychotherapy for years but had reached a plateau in her work. She intuitively knew she needed a different approach that could account for the nuances of her trauma history and complexity of her current presentation of symptoms. And though not exactly certain *how*, she felt certain that the place to begin her healing was "in the body." Nearly instantly upon meeting her, I knew I was in the presence of an artist. An artist mourning the contribution and interaction she once had with her life and the people in it—with herself and her creative spirit. An artist who more than anything wanted to be seen, and for her suffering to be acknowledged and validated. I felt confident that, at minimum, I could provide a space for her to be comprehensively seen in the way that her dynamic life deserved. She has since thanked me for this: "Thank you for seeing me. And for looking with me at *what I see*. I am deeply grateful to be seen and heard." Miriam once said that trying to explain to people what it was like to live with ME/CFS was like "screaming into a vacuum," preventing any audible cry from being heard, no matter how frantically she tried. This was terrifying to her. Not feeling seen or heard—and feeling invalidated, dismissed, or blamed—is such a common experience for so many trauma survivors.

The minimizing and diminishing response that so many survivors
are met with when they try to tell their story or seek help transcends
any one individual's singular response, as it is systemic in nature.
Jenn Turner, co-director of the Center for Trauma and Embodiment, has noted in a presentation that "we live in a world that
seeks to deny and silence experiences of trauma." Very often this
silencing is intentional, deliberate, and even coercive, most especially when trauma and abuse occur within the context of intimate
relationships that are meant to be safe. When these experiences of
trauma are denied, the abuser uses their power to decide what did
or did not happen. The experience of the survivor doesn't count.
It vanishes. And so often the survivor vanishes along with their
experience. Interestingly enough, this can also happen in more
subtle ways even in loving, safe relationships. Due to the socially
constructed nature of this response, the cyclical silencing that
has now become so deeply habituated and reinforced in our society is not always intentional. It's automatic. A knee-jerk reaction.
Unconscious, even. And unfortunately, sometimes *most* unintentionally in the context of loving relationships. It's why, on that early
gray morning on the Upper East Side of Manhattan when I called
my best friend to recount the tumultuous events of the previous
night before stepping down into the subway to let it all become a
faded memory, she clearly and definitively said to me: "No, no. You
weren't raped, Emily. You're okay." It's why both my mother and
husband said to me that it "*wasn't* postpartum depression" when I
was suffering so profoundly during the early days of my firstborn's
life. In these circumstances it's almost evolutionarily adaptive to try
and make the suffering go away. We don't want to see the people
we love in pain; and ultimately we do need to "move forward" to
survive. So we say "it wasn't rape," and it's just the "baby blues,"
and it will be okay. But even in the best of circumstances, individual experiences of pain, suffering, and trauma are being denied,
overlooked, generalized, or ignored. And this pain doesn't go away.
It makes its way into the cellular fabric of our being. Which is why
Miriam organically and viscerally knew: "*I strongly believe the place to*

begin 'recovery' for me is in the body." She knew that what she needed and what ensued in her healing process had both everything and nothing to do with me at the same time. It did have something to do with a neuropsychological function called interoception, a central tenet of TCTSY. The platform that TCTSY provides as "therapeutic scaffolding" for interoception to occur is nothing short of a work of art, in my mind. Miriam agrees. She is an artist, after all.

When Miriam used the metaphor "screaming into a vacuum" in relation to her desperate plea to be understood by the people closest to her, what accompanied that experience was a sense of terror. Terror not only of suffering to the magnitude and extent that she has, but terror in suffering *alone*. I don't think it's a coincidence, therefore, that when we experimented with TCTSY during our psychotherapy session for the very first time, she was overcome with fear. While lying on our backs on mats on the floor next to each other, we were experimenting with some simple actions of breathing and moving together. With palms facing up, Miriam was invited to open and close the palms of her hands, perhaps in a way that synchronized or matched the rhythm of her breath. I heard her take a few sighs, almost in desperation, and definitely in a way that felt distressing. Tears immediately started streaming down her face. When I asked what she was experiencing, she said she had become flooded with emotion and became "acutely aware of how scared I am." Although "hands-on assists" are not something we offer in TCTSY group classes, in that moment, I gently reached over to place my hand on top of hers. The moment my hand touched her, the tears increased but had a different quality to them. It was subtle, but there was relief present. A little space. Connection. A hallmark tenet of Judith Herman's unparalleled contribution to the trauma field is the idea that after the disempowering experiences of trauma, recovery can only truly take place within the context of relationship, never in isolation, therefore focusing on the "empowerment of the survivor and the creation of new connections."[4]

During another session, after a more active TCTSY sequence that offered Miriam the opportunity to feel her muscles and use her body in a way that she had not in a very long time, she said that this felt different from any other yoga she had ever practiced— that there was "something else happening here." One opportunity offered by integrating TCTSY into psychotherapy sessions is the ability to identify and verbalize connections/realizations made during the practice and expand upon them. We did this a lot. Sometimes Miriam would also send me emails several hours or even days after a session, drawing upon something she experienced in our work. At the end of this particular session, I said something along the lines of, whatever that "something else" she referred to may be—it was *hers*, and it didn't have to stay here: she could take "it" with her. She almost immediately froze up and verbalized that this was a very challenging sentiment for her to receive. While emoting, it was very hard for her to think about the idea of a "continuity of self," and a "sense of self" was not something she had felt connected to in a very long time. It was much easier to feel that the self could only exist when the conditions were right (in our case, doing yoga in the context of a safe relationship during her therapy session, at my office). She had lost, or perhaps never really had, an internalized sense of safety. Safety was dependent upon an external place or relationship. She once told me in reference to my office (more specifically, our relationship) that "this is where my hope lives." An email she sent following this session expanded upon the notion of the "continuity of self" and poignantly described her struggle.

Though neuroscience is an ever-expanding and evolving study, over the past decade there has been a significant advancement in the field's attempt to identify the location where this "continuity of self" may actually exist in the human brain (in the insular cortex, or more specifically the insula). Without branching off into a full-scale explanation of this neuroscientific discovery, let me share just a bit of what we've come to know about interoception. Neuroscientist Alan Craig, a leader in the study of interoception, has

I struggle with the intersection and lived experience of identity vs. self. I was a wife, caregiver, mother, daughter, friend, and respected colleague. Creatively generative. I felt competent and confident. I had a love affair with books and language. I was a documentary filmmaker. Working on the narrative meaning of other life stories. Who am I if my "self" is no longer in those roles? If I have lost the capacity? Who am I if the only witness to my whole self is my therapist? It is difficult and painful for me to feel the self when the fundamentals of identity are no longer true. This is the experience of "losing one's mind" and losing the physical experience of a continuity of self. Alone with illness. The body consequently becoming wholly unpredictable.

often described this phenomenon as representing the "feeling self." It is the process whereby external stimuli, or sensory inputs, are felt internally—perhaps through feeling sensation from external physical contact or movement, or from internal bodily cues (hunger, thirst, pain, temperature), both received as visceral, afferent sensory information from organized tissue in the body. What takes this phenomenon beyond the physiological ability to *notice* sensation is the concept of assigning "emotional valence" (do I want more or less of this?) to these sensations and deciding what *to do* with them. The feeling self informs and shapes our internal landscape, and it reinforces the fundamental ethos that *I exist,* that *I am.* It represents the internalized belief that one can respond to and make choices based on these felt sensory inputs. Furthermore, it suggests that one can act upon, manipulate, and even change sensations in order to take effective action and create different outputs. Neurophysiologist Clare Fowler speaks to this expanded definition of interoception: "As originally defined interoception encompassed just visceral sensations but now the term is used to include the physiological condition of the entire body and the ability of visceral afferent information to reach awareness and affect behaviour, either directly or indirectly. The system of interoception as a whole constitutes 'the material me' and relates to how we perceive feelings from our bodies that determine our mood, sense of well-being and emotions."[5]

Feelings drive behavior. We feel something and can then be driven to do something with and in response to that feeling. Each sensory input offers an opportunity for the generation of both a physiological sensation and a behavioral/emotional motivation or outcome. With interoception, a neuropsychological "stock taking" of sensory input occurs. But it's something a bit different from the traditional cognitive-behavioral question, "What does this feeling *mean* to you?" (i.e., the clichéd "How does that make you feel?" that every therapist ever depicted in the media asks their clients ad nauseum). Interoception instead asks the question, "What do you want *to do* with that feeling?" It brings us away from cognition and into visceral felt sensation. Out of the thinking mind and into the feeling body. Away from the stories and narratives of the past (often imprinted on the metaphorical broken record of neurophysiological conditioning), or the fears and what-ifs of the future, to the actual felt sensation of right now.

At the crux of "What do you want to do with that feeling?" lies the concept of agency. *Agency* is technically defined as "the capacity of a person to act in any given environment; the state of acting or exerting power, or to which an end is achieved; the capacity of individuals to act independently and to make their own free choices."[6] Consequent to her ruptured identity and sense of self, Miriam speaks of things feeling "penetrable" to her: "I am trying to be made whole. I need to find a way to return to owning myself." Interoception can strengthen belief and trust in one's own agency and existence. It also strengthens one's ability to interact and be in relationship with the world, to act upon the environment, and to choose and have choice. Neuroscientist Anil Seth and his colleagues believe that "as the embodied self is more fully realized through awareness of ongoing interoceptive interactions, two complimentary senses emerge: *presence,* one's connection to the moment, and *agency,* one's ability to effect change, which are both foundational in determining a person's sense of well-being."[7] Interoception, therefore, is not a process but an ability—or capacity, really—to use sensory experience to inform decisions, respond and make choices, effect change, and possess agency.

People with complex trauma have an under-activity or dysregulation in interoceptive capacitates, particularly in the insular cortex. David Emerson, the founder and creator of TCTSY, has suggested that to endure the chaos of complex trauma, survivors have had to become "exteroceptive geniuses," highly attuned and at times hypervigilant to external stimuli (which include relationships) in their environment, at the expense of developing or fine-tuning internal interoceptive capacities. If we overdevelop our exteroceptive capacity, we may be neglecting our interoceptive capacities. In our research and in scans of the traumatized brain, we have found that these interoceptive neural pathways have actually begun to physically atrophy. In TCTSY we are mindful of the altered interoceptive capacities likely present in the individuals we work with, and we make efforts to increase opportunities for engagement with these interoceptive pathways. During the practice of TCTSY there is a dynamic intersection and exchange of sensory stimuli (input) offered through physical shapes and forms, followed by opportunities for choice-making and response/action (output) based on those choices. Herein lies the concept that interoception is about not just one's relationship to and sense of their singular self but also their relationship to others and to the world. Interoception, therefore, is inherently *relational* in nature. We find purpose and meaning (and are instinctually driven to do so) through being in relationship with others or the world around us—by feeling like we are contributing in some way. We feel that we matter. Trauma takes away our instinct of purpose.

Miriam pointed out an additional aspect that made any recognition or interaction with a "sense of self" complexly challenging: her sense of self was so closely interconnected with her identity (not at all an uncommon experience), as evidenced when she said, "*It is difficult and painful for me to feel the self when the fundamentals of identity are no longer true.*" Here we may consider what, if anything, differentiates self from identity. *Self* can be defined as "a person's essential being that distinguishes them from others . . . a person's particular nature or personality; the qualities that make a person unique."[8] A psychological definition adds that the self maintains its continuity through time and place.[9] *Identity*, though similar, has more focus on the characteristics, beliefs, and roles of an individual, as well as the way one thinks about oneself and the way one is *perceived* by the world around them. It's a subtle difference, but I've always found the connection of identity to the roles that an individual may have in their lives—as a parent, partner, son or daughter, or in a career or vocation—as a helpful distinction from the self. These aspects of an individual are part of what helps define their sense of self, but the self can exist beyond these identities as well, since roles and identities will naturally evolve, shift, or even completely change over time. For Miriam, when she lost access to the identities and roles that defined her, including how she is seen and valued by others, her fundamental sense of self was lost as well. The two were so closely intertwined in her mind that one could not exist without the other. She was filled with such grief over the loss of her sense of self, and she concluded that any recognition or confrontation with the self felt traumatic, "like a blunt force to the chest." This is likely why, perhaps on an unconscious level, Miriam built up resistance to and protection from any self-acknowledgment/recognition. In fact it was much more comfortable for her to talk about how filled with self-loathing she was. Suicidal ideation, though not current for Miriam, has haunted her in the past. An email she sent after one of our sessions expanded upon this turning away from the self so eloquently:

I think what I felt/meant is that the self holds the loss. The truthful reality of all loss and trauma sustained. Recognition of the self, perhaps, is the shock of the trauma embedded that becomes potent and alive again. What happens when the self becomes traumatic? When the self and the conditions of my life become unacceptable? The sicker I've become, the less of a self I have. I vanish. I need others to feel seen.

The repetitive reliving and reexperiencing commonly described in experiences of trauma are so closely intertwined with one's self-awareness and self-possession, because the trauma, of course, and in fact, happened to the self. Miriam has spoken about waking up every day and "re-traumatizing" herself as she grieves and mourns her loss of herself, identity, functioning, success, agency, and effectiveness.

My entire personality has been altered. Small things overwhelm and confuse me. I make scheduling errors constantly. I can't maintain attention. I can't read. I can't stay on topic. My boundaries seem to have dissolved. The close friends and colleagues I had have been very scarce. I have become isolated. My relationships have all but faded away.

Miriam's fiancé left her at the peak suffering of her illness. There were elements of emotional abuse present throughout much of the relationship, particularly when Miriam began to psychologically decompensate. He always felt that she was exaggerating the symptoms of her illness.

No one is angry with someone for having cancer, but with ME/CFS, which is just as disabling, the patients are blamed. No one need exaggerate this illness. No one ever would. It is very much real. It is ruinous. I can no longer bear the anxiety of his [her ex-fiancé's] perpetual negation of this injury. I cannot be victim anymore. I will do anything to stop being his victim. He's dangerous to me, and I feel chronically helpless. In his denial, I've lost my humanity.

Miriam's feelings of rejection and abandonment are so profoundly pervasive as she states, "I was helpless and in danger and alone. My life was of no value." Trauma has impacted and injured nearly every relationship in Miriam's life. And the forced social isolation that she experiences from living with a chronic and disabling illness impacts her internalized sense of value and self-worth on a daily basis.

Because the cascade of illnesses that have led to my current health condition are invisible (brain damage causing functional cognitive impairment, mood disorder, PTSD), suffering feels/is both invisible and denied. I am necessarily alone in my experience. I have lost my sense of who I am and where to find myself in this period of my life. As compared to the narrative arc of cancer treatment which people embrace, support, dignify, and cheer on. One way or another it is expected to end. We fight and defeat. Or succumb after brave battle. No such meaning making narrative exists for the rupture of identity, or injury to the sense of self when chronicity, and invisibility define the experience. My "self" became marginalized in my psyche, just as "Miriam" became marginalized socially.

ME/CFS author Elisabeth Tova Bailey in *The Sound of a Wild Snail Eating* describes a "certain depth of [this] illness that is piercing in its isolation . . . the only movement is the passage of time. . . . Even if you are still who you were, you cannot actually fully be who you are. Sometimes the people you know well withdraw, and then even the person you know as yourself begins to change. . . . Illness isolates; the isolated become invisible; the invisible become forgotten."[10] Accepting herself as she is is very hard for Miriam. Many times during my facilitation of TCTSY, I offer the invitation to notice your body/self/breath "exactly as it is"—or "exactly as you are" in this moment, "just right now." Miriam once wondered if "radical self-acceptance" (her words) may be part of her healing— ultimately wanting to hold space for grief and joy simultaneously. When we practiced TCTSY together, there were moments when she was able to interact with self-acceptance and inquiry instead of self-loathing and rejection. I think another almost artistic quality of TCTSY is the space it creates for the fullest range and expression of the self, with and through sensation and connection (both physical and relational). Ultimately what emerges are new present-moment experiences that have never before existed—in the presence, witness, and validation of the cultivated and co-created safe relationship.

Herein lies another core tenet of TCTSY that we call shared authentic experience. When I said earlier that I had both nothing and everything to do with Miriam's healing process, I was speaking about shared authentic experience. What ultimately helped Miriam move away from isolation and toward connection was that I was able to show up as a fully human person in our therapeutic relationship. My presence was real and authentic. Genuine and vulnerable. I was a witness to and co-creator of new experiences and connections (both relational and neurological) with Miriam. Miriam has said that it is an "act of bravery to leave the trauma state." This state can entail complete overwhelm or a sense of inner vacancy, sometimes both at the same time. She describes leaving the trauma state as subsequently being an *open state*. And to be open and vulnerable is terrifying. "That said . . . I leave the trauma state when I'm here with you." Emerson often offers the idea that any moment of presence (or in TCTSY language, interoception) is "*not trauma*, no matter how brief of fleeting." Miriam and I were able to string together little moments of "not trauma," and we continue to weave that tapestry together in our work today. Nearly a year ago, leading up to the birth of my second son, we had the opportunity to "interoceptively take stock" of our therapeutic relationship to date, in hopes of building a sense of object permanency for Miriam to hold with her during my maternity leave. The idea that I would still exist; that our relationship would still exist, even in my absence.

I feel alive when I'm here. Because you dignify the process with the fullness of your own authenticity. And you can bring as many aspects of yourself to the table as are put in front of you. This is how an artist approaches her work. I am beyond grateful for the care and kindness you have shown me. You gave me an opportunity to express myself. And to feel love, safely. That is one of your gifts.

This very well may be the most touching feedback I have ever received from a client in my nearly two decades of therapeutic work in the field. As reaffirming and personally fulfilling as that feedback was, however, I'm not so certain this type of full witnessing could have existed were it not for the therapeutic platform that TCTSY offers.

I do not deny for one second the immeasurable value garnered from feeling truly seen and heard by another individual. But I do feel that, at minimum, TCTSY offered a concrete, empirically validated methodology that created a backbone for our relationship to scaffold from. It became possible to feel our own bodies in an authentically separate-but-together sort of way, which is something I've started to call *paralleled agency*. Being present to our own felt experiences through paralleled agency allowed us to more safely engage in relationship with each other. In addition, the invitational language and language of inquiry that are fundamental in TCTSY transcended the physical shapes and forms we explored together. This language became embedded in the therapeutic dialogue we had with each other in session, and in Miriam's own intrapersonal dialogue. She often said she could "hear my voice" outside of session "inviting" her to *notice* where she was, and to *explore/become curious with . . . maybe, perhaps, if she'd like, noticing* her breath in this moment, *exactly as it is . . . exactly as she is*. The language left an imprint. A subtle tone. The room for interpretation and personalizing in just saying the word "possibly" versus "it *is* this way" is significant. There's a bit more space and potential when words, concepts, and even physical shapes and forms are presented as invitational choices. There's an allowance for being self-directed, choosing for choice's sake, and being able to have a different experience from someone who may traditionally or historically hold a position of power, authority, and expertise (the therapist or yoga instructor). Emerson has spoken about how trauma doesn't make room for more than one person's experience. "To survive trauma, we have to either be defiant or allow ourselves to be subjugated to someone else and this will constantly be replayed in the relationship. When power is shared, being self-directed and able to have different experiences in and of itself is therapeutic."[11]

Just last week I teared up, as I have done a few times in my sessions with Miriam, when she jokingly called herself out for using "invitational language," noting the unconscious mirroring that has taken place in our work together and through our relationship. She said that love and connection (being in relationship) "create the possibility of possibility." The possibility of possibility—also known as hope. In this declaration, she allowed for and started holding her own hope. I will keep holding it too—for her, for myself, for trauma survivors around the world, and humanity at large—but I feel more confident that she doesn't need me to hold *all* of it for her. This speaks to how far she's come and how far we've come together.

In separate togetherness.

In paralleled agency.

Authenticity in Vulnerability

*Creating Connection with
Survivors of Forced Migration*

Elizabeth Ringler-Jayanthan

HAVING GROWN UP IN A small, rural community, I was fascinated by traveling the world, and my love of travel inspired my passion for working with international communities. I had never really left my community until I had the opportunity to travel with my high school Spanish club on a trip abroad, which helped ignite the fire in me to see the world and experience more of life outside of my small town. Having come from a working-class background, I also had a desire to help people who were denied access to resources such as education, and I wanted to find a way to be of service to others.

This led me to serving as a Peace Corps volunteer in Kyrgyzstan and an English teacher in rural China, and eventually to working with international populations in the United States, specifically with newly resettled refugees. For several years I served as a case manager at a local refugee resettlement agency and worked with clients from all over the world— Bhutan, Burma, Iraq, and many other countries. My primary role was connecting clients with employment opportunities, which involved coordinating interviews, helping clients complete job applications, and physically riding the bus with them to their first day of work. Soon I learned that their needs were far more expansive—clients often approached me with myriad concerns, including past and current traumas.

One particular family comes to mind. They had been refugees twice: once fleeing from their home country in the Middle East many years ago, and a second time when war broke out in the country of refuge. When they arrived in the United States, they had been in a camp for several months. The housing that our agency secured for them fell through at the last minute, and we put them up in a hotel for a week before securing new housing. The family was rightfully very upset and highly agitated in all our interactions during this time. We understood they were angry regarding the housing situation, but we didn't fully grasp that it could be a trauma response and how best to approach it. After about a year, the family was settled in stable housing and doing well, with all their children in either high school or college. Their healing was not possible until they first felt safe, and part of that was in having a safe place to live.

The concept of the triple trauma paradigm, which comes from the National Capacity Building Project, explains the trauma a forced migrant experiences during pre-flight, flight, and post-flight.[1] A forced migrant first experiences trauma that caused them to flee their home country, such as being targeted, discriminated against, or killed because of their ethnicity, race, religion, sexual orientation, political affiliation, or nationality. Layered on top of this is the trauma they may experience while fleeing, which may include violence such as rape, robberies, or exposure to the elements. And finally there is the trauma of being resettled in a new country, where the migrant may face language barriers, difficulty in adjusting to the new culture, discrimination, and loss of status and material wealth.[2]

Many of the clients I served often talked about their physical difficulties such as back problems, gastrointestinal trouble, and headaches. During a simple intake regarding employment background, some of the older Bhutanese men would reveal a past history of being imprisoned and tortured. In response to basic questions on employment, one client revealed that their father had been horrifically kidnapped and killed in his home country. It came as a surprise to me that these basic questions—not focused on mental health—could stir up people's traumatic memories and difficult content from their pasts. Some clients would tell me about violence they experienced in the United States, such as domestic violence or being robbed when walking home after work. As these issues came up in the case-management process, the conversation would move toward both helping the client make connections to resources and providing emotional support. I felt humbled that clients felt safe to come to me for help as these issues arose—but not equipped with the skills to provide the mental health support they needed.

Wanting to do more for my clients led me on my journey to become a mental health professional. In social work school, I learned about the mind-body connection to traumatic experiences, which helped me better understand how physical distress and trauma can be interrelated. One client in whom this stands out was a woman from Southeast Asia, a single mother with two young children and no other family in the United States. She had previously lived in a camp where many women were subjected to sexual violence. She often experienced severe gastrointestinal distress and would sometimes immediately vomit when coming into the office. The interpreter shared that she would only give one-word answers to any questions we asked. Despite seeing many doctors, she got no specific diagnosis or cause for the gastrointestinal problems. She struggled with maintaining employment and eventually moved to another state. In retrospect I have wondered if her symptoms could have been a trauma response and if I was just not equipped at the time to recognize the signs.

Though most resettlement agencies focus on meeting basic needs, such as securing housing and employment for newly arrived refugee clients, I had the unique opportunity to work at an agency that focused on refugee mental health. There I was moved by the ways the refugee community was supporting itself by training community members in recognizing and responding to mental health needs. They used Mental Health First Aid, which is a curriculum that is accessible to all community members, regardless of expertise in mental health, and has served as a useful tool to open up discussion on mental health in various refugee communities. The efforts made within the Bhutanese community to train in and respond to mental health have been particularly powerful given the number of Bhutanese refugees in the United States who have committed suicide, at rates much higher than the general population. The Bhutanese community has also integrated yoga classes for community members, an intervention that is accessible—and was familiar to the community before resettlement—and has also served as a form of social support. Many communities have begun implementing other forms of social support such as women's groups. In the Afghan community, for example, many of the women being resettled have lower levels of education, less work history, and feelings of isolation. Women's groups serve as a form of social support that helps the women acclimate to their new communities and dream for the future. These groups provide a space for women to improve their English, explore community college, look for jobs, and think about opening up their own businesses.

My social work program focused strongly on recognizing trauma and providing interventions, including yoga, for individuals who had experienced trauma. However, I did not see myself as someone who could offer yoga. I had never seen myself as athletic, particularly knowledgeable about yoga, or physically disciplined enough. Yet I met some individuals who were offering yoga to refugee clients and shattered the stereotype of what a yoga teacher "should" be like. These teachers shared with me the incredible connection that they were able to form with clients in this setting and how helpful it had been for clients facing very challenging circumstances. In social work school I had the opportunity to learn more about mindfulness techniques and yoga, which was an enormous help in better managing my own anxiety. When I was searching for a program that would be a good fit, Trauma Center Trauma-Sensitive Yoga (TCTSY) best met what I was looking for, and the philosophy resonated with me. I admired that TCTSY was not about perfecting the "right" movements but more about sharing an authentic experience with others, and it was intentional with the empowering element of choice for participants.

After finishing the social work program, I was inspired to bring new skills into my work with refugee populations. As a clinician, I have been greatly humbled to have had the opportunity to provide therapy to individuals from various backgrounds, including forced migrants, who have experienced trauma. I worked with a young survivor of torture from Venezuela, a refugee woman from Syria who experienced panic attacks, a man from Sri Lanka who spent many years in detention, and several foreign-born victims of human trafficking. These individuals were forced to flee their home countries due to being targeted for their political beliefs, their ethnic background or race, political views, or due to widespread war in their home country that caused a mass exodus. While these people experienced horrendous tragedy, they also demonstrated courageous strength in their resolve to move forward despite what they had faced. While I have seen many examples of this, one specific client comes to mind. She was a woman from the Middle East who experienced the unimaginable tragedy of losing her husband and children. Because of conflict in her country, she also lost the opportunity to become educated and could not read or write in any language. When she was resettled in the United States, she arrived on her own, without any other family, and started to learn to read for the first time in her life. She started working in her first job despite being the only one at her workplace who spoke her language and not being able to speak any English. She maintained her hope for the future and demonstrated her immense courage in facing these challenges. While she was separated from her children and did not know where they were, she maintained hope that one day she would be reunited with them. She maintained hope in her everyday actions by learning to take the bus, going to work, and coming to therapy.

Studies have shown that clinicians can experience vicarious post-traumatic growth from witnessing the progress of their clients, and I can say that I have been strongly impacted by witnessing people's capacity for resilience and hope despite the unimaginable suffering they have faced. It's difficult to put these feelings into words, but I have experienced a shift for the better in my overall worldview, and in my own capacity for growth.

One woman stands out, however, who I will call Grace. Grace was from a country in Africa and seeking asylum in the United States due to religious persecution. She had been living in a homeless shelter with her five children while she awaited her employment authorization and the decision of her asylum case. She was diligent in coming to her therapy appointments with me and brought along her small baby. While the Western notion of therapy was a new experience for Grace, she was open-minded and hungry to improve herself and her situation in any way that she could for herself and her children.

In my work as a clinician, I had learned of other professionals incorporating yoga with refugee clients. Knowing that many refugees experienced somaticized symptoms, I was hopeful that this could be useful for my clients. Although I myself was new to TCTSY, I began to incorporate elements of yoga into our sessions, including trying out TCTSY forms at the beginning or end of sessions. I told Grace that it was something I was learning and thought it could help her feel her body in a different way, which may help her feel more relaxed or simply be more aware of what she was feeling. We discussed how this was something we could do one-on-one together and she could also try on her own at home while her kids were at school. She said that she had heard of yoga but hadn't done it before. I was honest with Grace that this was new to me as well, and she was gracious and expressed her openness to try whatever I thought could be helpful. I felt a great responsibility to do the best I could and was grateful for her willingness to try something new.

We worked together in utilizing TCTSY in a way that made sense for her, starting out with just a few minutes at the beginning and end of our sessions together. I challenged myself to be vulnerable in admitting that I wasn't the expert even though I was the therapist, and she allowed herself to be vulnerable in trying something very new to both of us. Grace let me know when she liked a movement or form we did together, and we tried new forms that worked best for her. I offered Grace choices in different movements, and she expressed that some were relaxing or nice. After the TCTSY portion, I asked how the experience was; she told me what she liked or didn't like and how she may try it on her own at home.

When we first started the sessions, some movements felt a little strange or awkward for me, but Grace was very open to trying whatever I could offer, and that helped ease my fear. Sometimes during our sessions her baby would sit in her lap, and other times he would be asleep in his baby carrier; this required flexibility from both of us and helped strengthen the authenticity of our therapeutic relationship, in that it cultivated a sense that we were in this journey together. I offered Grace choice in the forms and choice in whether or not she wanted to do TCTSY that day. For someone who has limited choice in many areas of life, offering choices is important to maintaining the trust in the relationship. Grace reported that TCTSY helped her feel calm, even though the shelter environment was stressful.

Yoga practice became a part of our therapy routine, and Grace began to use some of it at home after her children went to school. Although I moved away from the city and was unable to keep working with Grace, I received an overjoyed text message from her a month or so after I left, letting me know that she had received her employment authorization card—a huge step forward for her. This was particularly significant as it allowed her the opportunity to start looking for jobs in the hope of moving out of the shelter, being more independent, and empowering her to think about the future.

I have also had the unique opportunity of serving as a volunteer for a group for foreign-born human trafficking survivors. The women in the group came from all around the world—the Philippines, Mexico,

Gabon, Ethiopia, Namibia, and many other countries. While the women spoke many different languages and came from different cultures, the women's group was a place for them to be in community with one another. The group became a safe place for them. Many of the participants remarked on how the women's group was their favorite part of the month, where they could be with women and feel calm and relaxed. One participant remarked on how it reminded her of what life was like in her home country.

The group utilized different types of interventions, including psychoeducation, art therapy, movement therapy, and TCTSY. This would be my first time facilitating TCTSY in a group setting. I had previously led processing groups as a therapist, but I had never led a group in a process that involved using your body. I was professionally vulnerable in a way that was new to me. In leading any group, there can be feelings of needing to be the expert, of possible judgment from others, and simply not knowing what to do next. I decided that I had to let go of that fear because what I wanted to share with them was worth the initial discomfort, and I couldn't learn without trying and releasing the fear. The group itself helped me get over my fear of facilitating TCTSY. Like Grace, these women were open to trying whatever I could offer, which helped when I felt like too much of a novice to lead a group in this practice.

The participants remarked on how they felt comfortable and relaxed. The women said that they had pain in the different parts of their bodies from the type of work they did during the day, which could involve standing for long hours or doing repetitive movements. Some clients shared that they would integrate some of the movements at home on their own. Most importantly clients were given choices, in the forms or movements that worked for them, and when and how to use TCTSY. Choice is of critical importance for this population who has had choice taken from them in so many ways, and specifically in relation to their bodies.

❦ ❦ ❦

In relocating to Washington, DC, I have been able to live one of my dreams: working at the national headquarters of one of the nine agencies that implement refugee resettlement across the country. In my role, I help individuals who work directly with the most vulnerable refugee populations nationwide. Anyone who works in the field of refugee resettlement, or with any immigrant populations today, will tell you that it is a very stressful time to be in the field. Federal policies regarding immigration and refugee resettlement are very hostile, and in some cases designed to intentionally inflict trauma. Many agencies, including one I previously worked for in Pittsburgh, have had to close because of the low numbers of refugees allowed to resettle in the United States. Not only does this create stress for staff, stretch resources, and create instability in one's job security, more importantly it causes refugee families, who may have spent decades in refugee camps, to wait even longer, with no clear path to refuge. Many refugee families have been divided, with some family members resettled in the United States (before the current administration enacted its policies) and some still stuck in camps—particularly people impacted by the so-called Muslim ban. Most recently, a new rule has been implemented that allows states and local governments to "opt out" of resettling refugees, leaving local resettlement agencies with the task of appealing to government leaders to support their programs.

Those working in resettlement have been going in to work every day, doing their work as usual, without knowing what the future will hold for the program and if there will be a program. This has prompted the question of what staff are doing for self-care. While this is always important for direct service workers, and particularly those who work with trauma, it has become more crucial with the new stressors. I was approached by a colleague who asked if I would be willing to lead a trauma-sensitive yoga class for staff. I agreed and began to lead a monthly class that integrated trauma-sensitive yoga and other self-care techniques. I was moved by the humility of the staff to be vulnerable with their co-workers in this space. For many people in this field, focusing on self-care is not a usual part of the job, despite working with individuals who have been severely traumatized and hearing stories of extreme trauma, including torture. There tends to be a prioritization of the impact to survivors, diminishing the real impact felt by service providers. This can be particularly true for case managers, who are often the first person a client may disclose their trauma story to. As a result there can be frequent turnover of case managers who experience burnout and vicarious trauma. Some case managers are also former refugees themselves and may become triggered by their own trauma history when hearing the stories of their clients. In coming together for the trauma-sensitive yoga classes, we helped lower the barriers that we place between ourselves in a professional environment and helped form a more authentic bond. I observed this through the staff's conversation after class, some expressing their own feelings of awkwardness in engaging in this type of activity, and others discussing things they integrate on their own at home and offering this to others in the group.

This is what I've gained most from trauma-sensitive yoga—and what I think people I've worked with have also gained—the ability to let go of pretense, to be vulnerable, to grow a richer sense of trust in others, and to be more at home with ourselves and others.

Just Two People in a Room, Trying to Have a Body

Relational Safety and Somatic Dissociation

Alexandra Cat

WE ARE DEFINED BY THE relationships we form.

For this reason, they can destroy us.

This is the tragedy of the human condition, the story of how we traumatize each other.

But it is also a redemptive tale, the story of how humans heal each other.

When we are seen and denied, we become *nobody*.

When another human sees us and allows us to be, we become *somebody*.

Darren emailed me toward the end of April 2017. He explained that he was attending psychodynamic group therapy, had attention deficit hyperactivity disorder (ADHD), post-traumatic stress disorder (PTSD), and possibly developmental trauma, was on medication for his ADHD, and his therapist had suggested that he try yoga. Darren had never done yoga before and was looking for some advice. He'd looked at my website and thought the Trauma Center Trauma-Sensitive Yoga (TCTSY) approach sounded interesting.

I offered Darren the option of a chat on the phone—a chance to ask questions and maybe build a sense of me. We followed up with a bunch of emails and eventually scheduled to meet in June. Since then we've met as often as Darren wants and I'm able— sometimes weekly and sometimes with longer gaps. We've explored headstands, handstands, and sun salutations, spent sessions lying on our backs, lifting our legs, and laughing at the weight of them. We've explored being out of breath and what to do next, and on occasion we've sat in chairs and noticed what it feels like to swivel our heads. Just two people in a room, trying to have a body.

> This was a very new experience for me. Up until this point, I had never felt safe enough to reveal my true intentions to anybody through fear of conflict or attack. I coped by having . . . different masks for any given situation. I was very much someone who could be whatever you wanted me to be at the expense of being myself.

The masks that Darren wore were protective. He had no reason to trust me or, as it turned out, anyone. People were a threat to be "managed," and Darren's strategy was to disappear behind screens of servility and vulnerability. He'd ask permission to look at me, ask a question, change how he was moving; he'd need to know if he was "doing it right," if he'd upset, angered, frightened, or repulsed me.

I would meet his questions with honesty—no, I wasn't angry with him, nor was I frightened, nor repulsed by him; yes, he could look at me and copy me, and no, there wasn't a technically right way to do the shapes. Rather, in each form I'd invite Darren to notice what he *felt* and let that guide his choices. Right alongside him, my gaze cast down, I would be exploring what I felt and allowing sensation to guide my choices.

TCTSY is a relational practice and not a self-practice. It is some-thing that we do with people; we do not leave, we stay alongside. In this sense TCTSY is fundamentally a practice of *not neglect*. But to offer a safe relational practice to a relational trauma survivor is no small task. A journey of the Self, through the Self, to the Self.[1]

"Having a body" is an entirely subjective experience—there is no right or wrong way to have elbows, or feet, or arms. Alongside this subjectivity of self is a basic human right: to explore oneself and build a life around what one finds—one's likes, dislikes, prefer-ences, and interests. When we deny someone this opportunity we erase them. In TCTSY we simply hold space for the opposite. An experience of *being*. An experience of *not trauma*.

> As each session progressed I would become more aware of my body. Just by allowing me to experience my feelings truthfully and honestly in an environment where I knew I was not going to be shamed or attacked was a very emotional experience for me.

Of course if safety and self have become defined by managing an outward threat, this particular yoga practice is not easy. To begin to attend to oneself after a lifetime of not is no small task. This is why, when clients are referred for relaxation, I smile an inner wry smile. All yoga practices are intended as a path of reconnection, and all states of yoga are, in one form or another, states of connect-edness. But to connect was a new experience for Darren, and it was sometimes a destabilizing and frightening experience. Initially he found neither himself nor safety:

Being a writer means . . . having to be curious about people and the world . . . for someone with symptoms of PTSD and a disorganized attachment it is a fucking nightmare. When sitting down to write I struggled to figure out what the motivation of character was and how to describe what mood they were in. The truth I feel is that I had no idea what I was feeling at any given moment or even how to authentically place myself in the world. . . . When trying to describe a character my mind would go blank which triggers my mother's critical voice . . . my mother's voice speaks to me whenever I try to learn a new skill or getting to know a new friend or partner. The voice will tell me that I am a fucking worthless piece of fucking shit and that I should die. Acting on this voice I will then sabotage any attempts to make my life better . . . she never saw me as something separate to herself. She was always trying to merge with me. I was never allowed to have any privacy from her . . . after I left home for university I was convinced that I was being filmed behind glass mirrors.

As the threat switched from the external—me—to these intolerable memories and intrusive voices, Darren switched gears. He put down his masks and picked up his dissociative tools. The white noise we all make would vanish and I'd *hear* Darren disappear.

The next time you're in company, try shutting your eyes and tuning in to how you know you're not alone. You'll hear a shuffle, a fidget, a sigh, an inhalation; you'll feel a quality of *presence*. Now open your eyes and notice all the varieties of ways this person expresses their unique, individual self. Perhaps in the way they style their hair or choose to sit, or the opinions, needs, and desires they express.

There are, however, occasions when we feel it safer to disappear ourselves. Sometimes this is as straightforward as being as quiet and as still as possible. On another occasion we might erase our self-expression and try to become more like someone else. Or we might become exquisitely attuned to anticipating and serving the needs of another. If our dread escalates we may fall into a dissociative shutdown state. An attuned facilitator will *hear* this. The sound of someone disappearing themselves.

In that silence with Darren, my commitment was to hold my nerve and hold our practice:

- An invitation to try a shape
- Options to notice sensation
- Options to explore making choices
- Options to make a choice based on what Darren was feeling

Each week the same shapes, the same invitations, the same choices. Each week the same pacing, the same intonation, the same rhythm. Each week walking the same fine line between containment and coercion.

This emphasis on predictability is the safety our clients rely on. After all, we work with people who expect to be blindsided by danger. But when people have checked out, it is less what we're saying and more how we say it that matters.

People say eyes are the gateway to the soul, but this is wrong. It's the voice. What we feel shows up there. My vocal presence told Darren I was alongside him whilst he felt what he felt, and that I wasn't going anywhere. My vocal presence is the rope I throw when he's dropped into a place of nameless dread. I never cut the rope.

Ironically it's around these more dissociative states that Darren has started to find the sensory footholds and handholds that *are* him. In every return to self, he's found a piece of self. Solid ground underfoot, a path to follow, a dependable, reliable, and predictable sensory self:

But if feeling is the foundation of identity, then knowing how to change one's feelings is the foundation of dignity and safety. Every time Darren and I walked the same path he discovered something new. Another way to be in a shape, a different way to move, a new way to change what he felt.

I was gradually becoming more aware of my body. I was repeatedly surprised by the fact that I had a body and that it is mine and no one else's. . . . After one session, I realised the awesome power of my legs and how much of a job they had had in keeping me upright. I was so elated by this experience I proceeded to take them off for a walk around London to make them work even harder!

Darren now knows he's someone who enjoys headstands and handstands and that they're a useful antidote to his anxiety and depression. He knows that he's someone who finds sun salutation physically demanding, that he can get overtired, and that he can choose to rest. Knowing that one can change one's feelings makes it slightly more tolerable to sit with them. This has had profound implications for the work Darren does in psychotherapy. After all, learning how to swim means that one doesn't have to drown!

For want of a better metaphor, I feel like a door has been opened. We have these amazing machines called bodies but often have no idea how to use them properly. It's not easy getting down on the mat for 20 minutes every day as life and the voices often get in the way. . . . I cope better than I did . . . I take my yoga mat to work so that I can take myself off when I feel anxious to do a few headstands. . . . As we've continued our work the many masks have started to slip away. I feel like I'm a hero on a quest to realize a more truthful and honest existence, making choices that are best for me . . . to be the hero of a journey that is very much my own and not someone else's.

TCTSY isn't an easy practice to describe. It's not a meaning-making practice like psychotherapy. It's not an affect-regulation practice like most somatic interventions. It's not a mindfulness practice like mindfulness-based stress reduction (MBSR) or its variants. It's not offered with the intention of building flexibility or strength or reframing the experience of touch. It isn't offered as catharsis, and it makes no assumptions about whether someone can feel or make choices about their experience.

Neti neti—not this, not that.

In this space something very profound happens. Just two people in a room, each of them trying to have a body. *Not* trauma. From this, atha yoga anushasanam—now, the teachings of yoga.[2]

MAKING CHOICES

My Road to Embodiment

Bailey Mead

IN OCTOBER 2008 I TOOK the first step on the long journey back home to my body. I remember sitting alone on my couch, stunned, until long after the sun went down. Shock eventually gave way to a slow rising sensation in my gut and chest that I hadn't felt in years and couldn't identify. This heavy wave rose steadily in my throat until I started crying, to my great surprise. Sobbing, loudly, for the first time in at least five years. The novelty of the sensation and the emotional release felt so strangely pleasurable and satisfying that I stayed with the sobbing as long as I could, exaggerating my sounds and letting the tears begin to bring something to life in me again after so long.

I had just met with my new therapist, a neuropsychologist, who told me the life-changing news that I had been taking the wrong medication for the wrong diagnosis for five years. She told me I was living with the effects of childhood and recent trauma, not bipolar disorder. Lithium, which I never wanted to take in the first place, which was keeping me from having children or hope or pleasure, and certainly from my creative inner life, wasn't even necessary.

I had not felt love in years. I had not cried in years. I could intellectualize my connections to others, but I could not actually *feel* love for my dog, my new nephew, or the man I was dating. I couldn't connect with nature or God. Everything felt just like everything else: not bad, not great.

My body was numb too. Gunshots rang out in my neighborhood almost every day, and I didn't notice them anymore. I drank myself to sleep most nights. My entire range of experience was lived on a continuum from "uncomfortable" to "kind of happy" and from hypervigilance to dissociation.

I felt I needed to be prepared for any number of horrifying things that had already happened and I therefore expected to happen again. For example, when I was twenty-six, I had been relaxing at home with trusted friends one Sunday evening when my parents, my roommate, and an assortment of other people burst into my apartment and all started chaotically telling me I had to get dressed and go with them. They wouldn't let me go to the bathroom by myself, and they lied to my friends about where they were taking me, so I was left to the devices and authority of these people who I had worked so hard to free myself from as a young adult. I was forcibly hospitalized, placed in solitary confinement after I walked outside to smoke, and then held and drugged against my will. It happened again about a year later. I was hospitalized against my will after being sexually assaulted by a group of five young men in an abandoned house on Detroit's east side. This time the staff threw my contact lenses in the garbage when I arrived. I am almost legally blind without them, and I was around legitimately dangerous people whose faces I couldn't make out. I was sexually assaulted by another patient. My medical records say I was "taken advantage of by a man with sociopathic tendencies." I was also sexually assaulted in the laundry room by a man on staff at the psychiatric hospital, all while blind and drugged into submission. I had been betrayed in ways I couldn't have imagined. I couldn't trust anything except the likelihood that it would happen again. I often ran through a scenario in my mind about how I would escape through my second-story southwest Detroit apartment window if they came for me again. I had a bag packed, a lock on the inside of the bedroom door, and a fire ladder.

I had surrendered to the idea that this was the best life I could expect. I gave in to the grim predictions that community mental health doctors and social workers had given me. All the books I could find on bipolar disorder reinforced the idea that unless I stayed on medication for the rest of my life, which in itself would cause serious health problems down the road, I would certainly get worse over time and possibly die decades early. I believed that as long as I got up, took those pills, and went to work every day, I was okay. I had been going through the motions of my life for five years, doing what was expected of me every day. I was surviving, but I wasn't living. I was performing, but I wasn't feeling.

I made a decision that night to reclaim my life, whatever that meant. I was afraid of what would happen if I stopped taking the medication. I read The Icarus Project's *Harm Reduction Guide to Coming Off Psychiatric Drugs,* and it gave me some tools and structure to work with. I spent the following weeks creating a detailed plan that enlisted the support of my two oldest friends and covered every possibility I could imagine. With the skilled support of my therapist and doctor, I slowly worked my way off of lithium and antidepressants and began to feel my way back into my body again.

Coming off of the medications was painful and intense. It's like being outside in the snow until your skin gets so cold it becomes numb, but when you start to warm up again the sensation becomes almost unbearable. Under these first layers of numbness and pain were more layers of intolerable sensation and old patterns of dissociation. Like a lot of people I know, I grew up in an alcoholic home, I was sexually assaulted as a child and as an adult, and I have dozens of stories about the everyday kinds of harm working-class girls encounter when there is never enough money and no one is paying attention to or protecting them. I had been surviving a long time before I ever took lithium, and it was a long road to get back to myself.

As I met with my therapist week after week, she created a safe, consistent container where I could explore my slowly thawing bodily sensations, emotions, and memories. She told me about the work of the Trauma Center in Boston, whose studies were demonstrating yoga as a treatment for complex trauma. At that time, there were no Trauma Center Trauma-Sensitive Yoga (TCTSY) facilitators in my area. We talked about me finding a yoga class so I could experiment with how yoga might help me stay present in my body without uncomfortable or intolerable sensations. This sounded good, but I faced so many obstacles to actually going to a class.

For starters I was uncomfortable in my body. I was sure I would be the biggest person in the room. I was self-conscious about my feet and didn't want to go barefoot. Although I was desperately trying to quit, I was embarrassed to go into a yoga studio smelling like cigarettes or coughing like a smoker. I was worried about what to wear and whether my body would stay in my clothes while we moved through the poses. I also felt like I was outside of my body, or in my head, a lot of the time. In fact, my early memories of practicing yoga at this time are all from a bird's-eye view, rather than from my own internal perspective.

Even though I had been practicing yoga on and off for more than a decade, I had only taken a few classes in studios. There were very few in my area at that time, and most of them were located in the wealthy suburbs. I had been to two studios, but they were not places I wanted to go again. The first was a Bikram studio. Practicing in the heat made me feel woozy and overheated. The backbends made me nauseous, and the mirrors made me feel ashamed and disembodied. The second studio was one of several in a local chain that featured classes with rock-and-roll music, many of them taught by male teachers who wore jeans but no shirts. As an assault survivor, that felt more like a college party than a yoga class.

I kept asking and searching around, but I didn't find anywhere I felt comfortable going. My therapist gently encouraged me over the next year or so, and I finally worked up the courage to try a studio in the next city over, about thirty minutes from my house. The website was intimidating, with Sanskrit characters, Hindu art, and quotes from the Bhagavad Gita. I heard from some friends about a free community class there on Saturdays, and I decided to try it. The ashtanga-inspired vinyasa class was intense and difficult, but it was the first time I had felt anything that powerful and positive in my body in a long time. I knew after the first class that I wanted to keep practicing with this teacher. I was moved by his clear authenticity and dedication to the principles of yoga. Born and raised a Brahmin in India, he lived simply in a modest home within walking distance of the yoga center, and he personally taught thirty classes each week. His approach was authentic and grounded in tradition, which felt safe and accountable compared to the haphazard experiences I'd had in the other studios.

I signed up for an introductory month of yoga and was determined to come to as many classes as I could. The practices were extremely challenging, and my muscles were painfully sore almost all of the time. This in itself was a kind of embodiment, keeping me constantly aware of my physical body in the present moment at times when I would normally forget I even had a body. I loved the enduring calm I felt for the rest of the evening after a class. I had been living with anxiety and discomfort for so long that it was a relief when my hypervigilance would settle down and I could relax enough to go to sleep.

After attending vinyasa classes for a while, I decided to try a restorative class. The vinyasa classes moved so quickly that all of my attention was on moving my body fast enough to keep up with everyone else and trying to somehow catch my breath. There was no opportunity to feel anything. Restorative yoga was another thing altogether. I was able to hold myself still through the forward bends and twists with some restlessness and discomfort, but when we moved into viparita karani, or "legs up the wall pose," and I felt myself lying on my back in the dark among strangers, with my eyes closed and my legs up in the air, my whole body started to shake and I felt like I couldn't breathe. I was having a panic attack. It didn't occur to me to mention this to my teacher. I tried to just breathe my way through it and get out of there quickly.

All the classes began and ended precisely on time. If I was one minute late, I would find the front door to the yoga center locked. I appreciated knowing what to expect, even if it meant I would sometimes miss class if I ran into traffic on the freeway. I drove for thirty minutes to get there, so if I was late, I would often walk over to a coffeehouse and wait for the next class to start an hour and a half later.

My teacher made a ritual of locking the door to the street, entering and closing the door to the practice space behind him, and then taking his seat to face us just inside the room. He was always the first to stand and leave when our practice ended. Then he would wash his hands and take a seat in the entryway. This consistency helped me feel less hypervigilant and more able to focus into my own body knowing that no one was coming in once class started. My things were safe in the entryway, and the practice space was secure. Facing the door while we practiced also helped me relax. I had been taken off guard and harmed several times in my life while I was sleeping or resting, and I was pretty much always alert and ready for something to happen out of the blue or for someone to come out of nowhere, especially when I started to relax my body. It took some time, but the unfailing consistency of the class format eventually helped me feel comfortable enough to begin to soften my gaze, close my eyes, and turn my attention inward toward the felt sense in my own body.

There was a rule about not talking in the actual practice space. I appreciated this because it gave the room a sense of being safe and sacred in some way. It gave me some privacy. It gave me the choice of whether to sit on my mat and look around at my surroundings or close my eyes and focus inward on my own body, which felt increasingly possible over time. It made the environment feel predictable, and I was able to begin to notice my own experience because I didn't need to engage directly with the people around me.

Beyond the ritual of entering and exiting the space, classes always began and ended in the same way, and the sequences were variations of the same theme. Each class would begin with several minutes of silent sitting before chanting Om. We always began with cat/cow stretches, then downward-facing dog and sun salutations, before moving through a series of challenging standing poses, followed by seated forward bends, twists, backbends, inversions, and savasana, or rest. We sat in silence together again at the end of class.

I've never met another yoga teacher who offers a class every single day, let alone five times every single day. I cannot imagine the energy required to do this. It was a gift that allowed me to keep coming back and experiencing my body in a consistent space, day after day, over the course of two years. I felt physically uncomfortable around most men, so this teacher was an unlikely choice, but he had impeccable boundaries around sexual energy with me. It was the first experience I could remember of receiving physical touch and energetic support from a man without a sexual undertone.

Between my weekly sessions with my therapist and four to five yoga classes with the same teacher each week, I began to trust and feel grounded by my relationships with these two people who felt authentically invested in my well-being. There was also something about the community of yoga practitioners that helped me feel connected, even though our time together was spent mostly in silence. My practice at the yoga center also connected me back to my own neighborhood when I began sharing rides with a woman I met there who lived down the street from me.

Over time the intensity of the classes allowed me to practice staying with strong sensations in my body, by my own choice, while simultaneously finding stillness and peace in the center of the intensity. I noticed that I was sometimes able to find moments of complete presence during difficult conversations or frustrating meetings at work. I found myself able to stay present and alert while walking from my car to my apartment in the dark instead of feeling overcome by anxiety and zoning out. I occasionally began to notice sensations of constriction or expansion in my body while moving though my days, giving me present-moment information about the people or situations around me.

These benefits were so tangible that I was able to ignore or tolerate some other things about the practice that were not as beneficial. I know now, as a facilitator of Trauma Center Trauma-Sensitive Yoga, how many of these things actually led me away from my body and unintentionally replicated trauma and oppressive power dynamics.

The classes were very structured, moving in sync at a predetermined pace. For the duration of each class, my teacher played a recording of his own ujjayi breath like a metronome while the class moved and breathed in unison. I often had a hard time keeping up with the class. I have asthma, and my breath was not very deep or steady. During every practice, I found myself skipping or doubling up on my breath in order to keep up. This lent itself to a disembodied practice where I, and probably others, was trying to appear to be in sync rather than attuning to my own body and breath. The practices were so fast and physically challenging that I was almost always in some kind of pain while practicing and in the days afterwards. I used pounds of epsom salt, arnica, and tiger balm during those years. I assumed the pain was because I was not strong enough, but in later years I encountered embodied teachers who helped me understand that my own breath should guide my movement. As my practice has shifted to one that provides me with grounding, presence, and regulation, I have rarely experienced pain after practicing asana.

After practicing at the yoga center for about a year, my teacher asked me to join a group of four other students who were going to train with him that year to become yoga instructors. I paid my tuition and began spending much more time at the center. Before I joined this group, my teacher had been neutral but compassionate toward me in his adjustments and in our discussions. Once I became a formal student, he was much more critical of me during our training and during regular yoga classes. At some point, he began poking my abdomen as a cue to engage those muscles. My grandmother used to do this to me as a kid. She would poke me out of the blue in front of a group of others and say "TTI!" which meant "Tuck your Tummy In!" As a child it felt embarrassing, invasive, and shaming. As an adult I wrote this about it in my journal: "I know I need to strengthen my core. My teacher has been poking his finger in my belly lately. Maybe I can figure out some way to work on it." He talked about body size in ways that I interpreted to mean he felt I needed to lose weight. He also set limits on the kinds of foods we were to eat during our eight months of training, and he was unhappy with me for bringing tempeh in my lunch because it was fermented.

His method of instruction was primarily through hands-on adjustments and commanding language, giving succinct verbal cues as he moved systematically through the room from person to person, giving adjustments. On one hand, there was an aspect of human connection and touch that alleviated a profound loneliness I felt much of the time. On the other hand, I felt obligated to accept, and even be grateful for, these adjustments, which sometimes encouraged me to move too far into a pose, causing pain and injury. I now know that trauma survivors are often unable to say no, even if we mean it.

In general, whether because I had been socialized to please the teacher or because he was always pointing out ways I could be just a little better, I always felt like I was performing. Sometimes I would be in so much discomfort appearing to hold a complicated pose that I would go somewhere else in my mind until it was over just to endure it. There was nothing in the mode of instruction or the culture of the studio that encouraged exploration or inquiry into my own experience of a pose. It was more like an army practicing drills in sync, toward perfection. Although my teacher would never call himself a guru, he held power in a way that positioned him as an expert who had great influence on his students' lives. I believe wholeheartedly that his intentions were only the highest, and I am eternally grateful for the time I spent practicing with him. It has transformed my life. Yoga is an ancient science that offers profound healing and transformation, but a cloud of avidya, or ignorance and misunderstanding, hangs over the yoga community about the role that power dynamics play in either healing or perpetuating trauma, and about the ongoing impact of trauma on bodies. This keeps the most well-intentioned instructors from upholding the primary ethic of teaching yoga: ahimsa, or non-harm.

§ § §

After practicing with this teacher for two years, I moved several hours away and began looking for other opportunities to further my practice and education. During this time, yoga seemed to explode in terms of people taking 200-hour teacher trainings, opening studios, and then immediately training other people to be teachers in order to remain profitable. It felt more difficult to find experienced, authentic teachers grounded in tradition. I found a studio whose lineage offered a nuanced understanding of the energetic practices of yoga and began to practice there. Trauma survivors are experts at sniffing out inauthenticity, and my experiences there seemed to indicate that this studio valued profit over relationship. Almost every interaction felt transactional, encouraging me to attend a retreat in some other country, purchase private lessons, or attend another teacher training. I often felt that the instructor was putting on a performance and expected adoration. We were encouraged to push past our discomfort and to smile big fake smiles through difficult poses. We were often surprised with partner yoga poses, where we were to turn to the stranger next to us, get very close with them, and then touch them or trust them to physically support us in a pose. Although I learned much about pranayama and subtle practices that helped me along my path to embodiment, I eventually could not attend classes there anymore because I felt on guard every time I tried.

After several more years of practicing mostly on my own, I met a teacher whose practice was wildly different from anything I had experienced before. It spoke deeply to my experience as a woman and a trauma survivor. She has studied with some of the most respected and embodied teachers in the world for more than two decades. She holds a space that is distinctly feminine and deeply respectful of yoga's teachings and traditions while being critical of traditional yogic power dynamics. She herself is a trauma therapist and ayurvedic practitioner, in addition to being a teacher of teachers. She leads practices that encourage practitioners to feel into their own bodies and to decide to move in ways that break the "rules" of alignment and static holds. She moves through the world in such an authentically embodied way that it feels liberating to spend time with her. I took every opportunity to practice with her, which was only about once a year because she lives in another part of the US. When she offered a 500-hour teacher training, I jumped at the chance to meet with twenty-six women from all over the world for five eight-day gatherings over the course of the year. The experience of being in this circle of women and working in such a deep way together over time was transformative in itself. One of the five gatherings was focused on awakening shakti, female embodiment, sexual trauma, and the ayurvedic approach to menstruation and menopause. This may have been the most profound and transformative experience of my life so far. I focused my studies on trauma-sensitive yoga that year, reading everything I could find on the subject, including David Emerson's book *Overcoming Trauma through Yoga*. I began to shift my own teaching in some ways, including backing off from hands-on adjustments, creating safer practice spaces, and using language that encouraged choice and present-moment awareness of the body. I also created a presentation to share with other yoga instructors and offered it to several 200-hour teacher trainings and gatherings of yoga teachers.

A few years later, I had the opportunity to complete a 300-hour training with the Center for Trauma and Embodiment and become certified as a TCTSY facilitator. This experience provided me with a nuanced scientific understanding about how trauma works in our bodies. The fact that TCTSY is grounded in feminism, neuroscience, trauma theory, and attachment theory made me feel like I have finally found my home in yoga. It is a way of practicing and leading that does not cause harm. It has changed me as a survivor and a facilitator, and the effects have expanded into many areas of my life.

One of these areas is choice-making. Trauma and oppression take our choices from us. For me, letting others make choices about my body and my life had been a matter of survival. I was "easygoing" and rarely voiced a strong opinion, even if I had one. What I learned about sex as a young person was that my desires and choices didn't matter and that if someone wanted to do something to my body, it was safer to let them do it even if I wanted something else. Practicing TCTSY encourages us to make choices in each moment about what we do or don't want to do with our body, and this feels revolutionary. It has helped reinforce the fact that this is MY body and no one else can tell me what to do with it. In the beginning, it felt so powerful to make these choices in the context of yoga practice, and then it began to seep into other parts of my life and the effect has been transformative. I started to speak up about conditions in my workplace that weren't working for me, like doing detailed editing work in an open-office environment, and I chose to work more often from home. I began to feel less self-conscious about making everyday choices that contradicted others' desires, like choosing to eat what my body desires or needs instead of what someone else offers me. I'm better able to say no, even when others are disappointed. Because I am using phrases like "one possibility is . . ." and "maybe . . ." when facilitating yoga practice, I find that flexibility and openness are spreading to the way I speak to myself and others. I found myself writing "*maybe* work on the budget" on my to-do list one day, which is a big shift from my habit of using that list to drive myself through the day and feeling like I come up short when I never accomplish it all.

Another integral part of TCTSY is sharing power and breaking down the traditional power dynamics between teacher and student. Judith Herman asserts that "no intervention that takes power away from the survivor can possibly foster her recovery, no matter how much it appears to be in her immediate best interest."[1] In the context of yoga practice, subtle shifts in language that offer choice and invitation instead of commands really do create a shift in power. I notice it acutely now when I take a regular yoga class. For example, I was recently on vacation practicing with a new teacher, and even though I am conscious of trying to choose for myself, the commanding language and the urge to prove my ability and knowledge to the new instructor kept creeping up. When I began to move in my own way, she corrected me as if she knows more about my bodily experience than I do. The experience of bringing consciousness to power dynamics has, and still is, creating shifts in my relationships with colleagues, doctors, my partner, and any authority figures I encounter in the world. In my work life, I began to speak up clearly about disempowering and contradictory practices. I also began to talk with my partner about subtly coercive patterns in our relationship, and I'm working on getting more comfortable with conflict. I was diagnosed with a hyperthyroid condition, and when the doctor insisted that I had to have my thyroid removed immediately and that I was being "emotional" because I didn't want to do that, I left his office. I sought out a functional medicine doctor who treated me with respect and dignity and empowered me to heal my gut and autoimmune condition through diet and supplements. The act of healing my gut, or innermost physical boundary, has begun to radiate outward into my ability to create boundaries in all parts of my life. It is restoring my voice, my agency, my courage, and my freedom.

As a facilitator, learning to share power while being authentic feels like such a relief. I finally feel like I know how to be in right relationship with others, without having to be an expert on their experiences, without attaching to outcomes, without trying to influence or move them in any way. I can simply show up as one human being with another, curious about the other's experience and keeping my focus on my own experience. This has helped me drop the pretense of being an expert in yoga or anything else in life, and there is such freedom in being humble and present instead of needing to appear to have it all together in every situation.

The yogic practice of self-study has been an invaluable tool for me in turning my attention inward and learning what works for my body rather than persisting with what works for other bodies. TCTSY emphasizes interoception, or noticing internal bodily sensations, and this has helped me turn inward and ask myself not only how I feel in any given shape but what effect it is having on my body. In traditional yoga classes, the instructor often says where a person should feel sensation and how it should feel, but everybody is different and may experience the same thing differently from day to day. Part of trauma is having our experience decided for us by someone else, and part of healing is reclaiming that ability for ourselves. By studying myself and my reactions to different yoga forms and practices, I have very slowly been able to build a practice for myself that encourages balance and calm. Although it's still sometimes a challenge, this self-study has given me the ability to have boundaries around what I do and don't want to do as a student in a yoga class. For example, I learned that shoulderstand and plow pose constrict my throat in a way that causes panic and constriction in my body. Although it still feels difficult sometimes in a traditional class to do something different from everyone else, I am now able to modify or sit these poses out. I spent so many years in my head with no awareness of what I was feeling in my body. By repeatedly turning inward and bringing attention to my internal felt sense, I am becoming more at home in my body and more trusting of myself and my ability to identify my own needs and care for myself from moment-to-moment. I have been able to show up for myself more consistently, using my daily practice as a way to create a more secure and trusting attachment with myself. This has allowed me to expand my world in ways I never thought possible, such as traveling to another country on my own, knowing I can care for and trust myself to meet my own needs.

I am moved to my core by the compassion and dedication that compelled those at the Center for Trauma and Embodiment to work for so many years to develop and demonstrate this model that addresses complex trauma with such integrity and dignity. It has led me home to my own body, in community with others, in the present moment. We all deserve this experience of being at home in our bodies, and I am honored to be empowered to share this gift with others.

A Feeling of Wholeness

Yoga with Refugee Children Living with Disabilities

Jemma Moody

> *We use our minds not to discover facts but to hide them. One of the things the screen hides most effectively is the body, our own body, by which I mean, the ins and outs of it, its interiors. Like a veil thrown over the skin to secure its modesty, the screen partially removes from the mind the inner states of the body, those that constitute the flow of life as it wanders in the journey of each day.*
>
> —ANTONIO R. DAMASIO[1]

HAVE WE LOST THIS CONNECTION with the interiors of our bodies? And at what cost? How do we live in a body that we are told is "broken" or "fragile" or "underdeveloped"? And how can we explore the wholeness of our bodies in order to live out the wholeness of our lives?

We each navigate the world in a body interacting with our environment, with our daily experiences, wandering in the journey of each day. Within this vessel of our being we carry our sense of self, our connections and relationships, and all the complexities of what it means to be human. And what I have found over the years is a curious awareness of what happens when we bring these bodies together, when we share space, when we move and breathe in unison together. What is it that happens when we begin to interact with our world through our felt experience of it? What does this mean for our relationships, for our sense of self, and for our path toward recovery?

When I first stepped into the world of social work over a decade ago, I was asked to sit with a young woman who was seeking asylum in Australia. She had survived sexual abuse, and I was asked to simply sit with her. We did not share a language, just a knowing smile of acknowledgment and support. And we sat together for well over an hour while she waited for her counselor to meet with her. This was a moment that shone a light on what it meant to connect bodily, to interact beyond language. And over the years this is where my career has taken me, toward an understanding of the importance of working with the body and toward a passion and curiosity for how we can build connections and relationships where we lack a shared language and where we are painfully aware of the imperfections of language, even if it were to be available.

I felt the pull to support refugee populations from the very first days of my career in social work. This displacement, dislocation, separation, and loss somehow tugged at the very core of my values. Learning of the plight of refugee populations worldwide made me question my privilege and luck to be born a white, middle-class, Australian woman. At first came guilt for this privilege and then an uncertainty of how to move forward and face it.

I left Australia. I traveled and tried to learn languages and understand cultures and consider my place in all of it. And time and again, I found myself working with refugee populations, displaced communities from Palestine to India to Turkey to Greece. My roles often changed depending on the context and the need, but I held space for these bodies, our bodies, to connect, move, and explore the experiences we shared. While working within a movement therapy program with Syrian children in Istanbul some years ago, I decided to delve into the world of yoga and complete my training. I witnessed how movement offered these children opportunities to explore their bodies, to find new ways of moving, and to express themselves nonverbally. Yoga had been a part of my life and my self-care practice for a number of years, and I saw how it could open a door to embodiment, really living in one's body, as well as an opportunity to connect nonverbally and to build, through movement, a sense of belonging. My yoga teacher training offered me a chance for a deeper exploration of my own body and an opportunity to facilitate moments of movement, rhythm making, and flow with other bodies. I knew at this point that this journey would take me to trauma-sensitive yoga, having crossed its path in Australia with sexual assault survivors a few years earlier. I had witnessed the healing nature of trauma-sensitive yoga with sexual assault survivors, I had met participants and heard their stories of recovery through their bodies, and while working with these children in Turkey I felt how trauma-informed movement may offer paths to healing for these remarkable young people. Essentially, Trauma Center Trauma-Sensitive Yoga (TCTSY) was my goal, my point of focus toward incorporating bodywork as a tool for healing and recovery into my social work practice.

By the time I found myself facilitating TCTSY, I had been working with non-English-speaking populations for the better part of a decade. I was interested in language, the words we choose, and how we point to an embodied experience using language in all its imperfections. Describing a felt experience in one's body is not universal. What I sense as "tingling" may be experienced by another as "vibrating" or "itching." To describe a sensation of "pressure" or "contact" may feel more like "tension" to someone else. Our language is subjective, and I feel that descriptions of language within my practice have led to confusion and at times guilt or a sense of failure from my clients who may feel something different, or perhaps not be aware of sensations at all. These observations and experiences have sparked a keen interest in exploring and navigating this world of embodiment without language, or at least with minimal language, because often that is all I have had in my practice. I began to ask myself how we may invite a felt experience of the present moment without words, how we could offer opportunities to take action based on our bodily experience without saying so.

For me, two key components of TCTSY have been central to
exploring these nonverbal interactions—choice-making and taking
effective action. Choice-making involves providing participants
with opportunities to decide how they would like to arrange their
body, offering different options for movement, perhaps different
points of focus where a participant could rest their awareness. And
then the participant may take effective action. They may be aware
of sensations in their body, how their body feels, perhaps what
it needs in any given moment. Participants can then take action
based on these sensations, choose how they interact with a form to
meet the needs in their body. I have been exploring a range of ways
to do this with greater and lesser success in different contexts and
with different populations. I have trained and used interpreters in a
number of settings in an effort to be accessible and to connect with
the individuals and groups as much as possible. When language is
imperfect, this translation, not only through words but also across
cultures, has at times created a barrier for me. This may be because
of the intricacies and details of the language itself; it may also be
because of the time it takes to work across two languages. Especially
with children, my experience has been that fewer words are better.
We can hold space and interact in a more authentic way without
describing what is or should be. Connecting with children in my
work has always been more felt, more bodily. A smile, of course,
communicates a lot. So does crouching down to a child's line of
sight, meeting them where they are, and so does sitting by their side
when they are distressed or disconnected. Through my presence,
through being available at the community centers and schools I
have worked in, I have sought to position myself as a visible and
accessible member of their community.

I have been privileged to have the opportunity to work with
the Syrian community in Turkey on a number of occasions, most
recently in Izmir where I was invited to share TCTSY with refugee
children living with disabilities. My role opened up opportunities
to facilitate group TCTSY sessions as an adjunct to children's ongoing physiotherapy programs. Some of these children were accessing

physiotherapy in their recovery from war-related injuries and others for physical disabilities from birth. The children's experiences were remarkably diverse, some living with paraplegia, others with an amputated limb, one young girl living with brittle bone disease, and a number of children with cerebral palsy. This diversity created such beauty in our sessions, so many possibilities for movement and for building connections through supporting one another and witnessing each other's strengths and resiliency. Collaborating with a physical therapist in this context allowed for the addition of mental health support to their recovery, with an emphasis on choice-making and sharing power. It wasn't common for these children and their families to access mental health care. Mental health care is often highly stigmatized within these communities, but beyond this, the families and individuals I worked with needed to have their basic needs met, to earn a living, to put food on the table and a roof over their children's heads. Coupled with the ongoing questions, bureaucracy, and uncertainty of the refugee determination process, mental health care was not a priority. Survival came first. So the question I raised was how to bring mental health to where they are, how to make it not only accessible but also appropriate and supportive. TCTSY offered that bridge, that step just beyond physical care that the individuals I worked with were open to exploring and experimenting with. It was about providing space for these children to have agency, to take action based on the needs of their bodies in that very moment. During this work we explored feeling whole, feeling unbroken. Whether they were living with disabilities from birth or injuries related to war, our sessions explored what it meant to feel complete. My biggest challenge was finding language, verbal or nonverbal, to invite participation and exploration of their bodies, and thus their lives.

Bringing yoga cards and props to the sessions offered visuals for the children to explore. Yoga cards showed a range of forms the children could experiment with, from forward folds to twists, breathing practices, and restoration forms. When the children entered the session the cards were displayed for them to look over, wondering what they might feel like doing in their bodies on that day, how they might make a particular shape, and what props they might incorporate into their practice. They chose the forms they wanted to experiment with using the cards, and then as a group they decided on the sequence. I regularly took pinwheels and feathers for the children to observe their breath with. These props acted as a bridge into noticing their breath in their body. One of the rooms we practiced together in was a preschool classroom that included a number of small chairs as well as soft toys that could act as cushions. I laid blankets on the floor, creating a space, a container perhaps, for our practice, and the children chose where they wanted to arrange themselves in the room. This could be based on proximity to me, to the other children, to the chairs, to the door— it was their choice. Then as we moved through the sequence they had created, this is where I saw the beauty of the practice unfold. The children worked together and experimented with adaptations and variations to meet the needs of their bodies. They could move the chairs around, perhaps leaning on a chair for support, perhaps holding a chair in a forward fold. How did this prop impact their experience in their body? Did it create a new or different shape? The children moved props for each other, they shared the pinwheels and feathers as they noticed the impact their breath had on the outside world, and I felt that as we moved and breathed together, creating rhythms and attuning to each other, we created a safe space to belong and to explore creativity and play based on our bodies, as they are. During these sessions the children navigated the very flow of their lives. It wasn't about survival or taking care of siblings or parents. It was about practicing being, perhaps different ways of being, in this body.

I recognize and acknowledge the very privilege I have been afforded for my life to never have been about survival. This privilege, however, was never named; it did not exist in my vocabulary until I left

Australia and met it face on. I have always had the privilege of freedom of movement, although until spending time in countries where this was not a universal right, I did not truly know this privilege. I have visceral memories of realizing this privilege while spending time in the West Bank in the Palestinian Occupied Territories many years ago. I would pass through checkpoints regularly, being ushered through cage-like structures toward turnstiles and military personnel checking visas and passports. With my blue Australian passport in hand I knew I would be allowed to cross, while the locals traveling alongside me never knew if their passage would be restricted on any one day. I had been told that if any conflict started all I needed to do was hold my passport up in the air and I would be removed from the situation. What a privilege this is, that by nature of the land I was born on, I could avoid harm and discrimination. My memories of this experience, and many others in countries and regions where basic rights are afforded only to a privileged few, are filled with sadness for my colleagues and friends who still do not have access to these rights, whose daily lives continue to be about survival. What I found in my work with refugee children has been the value of creating space for their experiences not to be about survival. To carve out moments in our shared experience together when we could explore the present in an environment that was safe, welcoming, and non-judgmental, where they are free to move their bodies, to navigate their experience in their bodies, to wander in the journey of that moment without limits or expectations.

When we work alongside refugee communities, we almost inevitably meet people in the midst of trauma or displacement. We meet them in the midst of uncertainty and doubt. The refugee process is long, it is cumbersome, and it is full of uncertainty for the future. My experience has been that this is one of the hardest aspects to bear—How long will we be here? When will it end? Where will we be sent next? All agency, all power and choice-making, is taken away.

What TCTSY offers in these contexts is in fact a wholehearted focus on the present moment, because this is all we are interested in. My role therefore was to navigate and nurture space in this very moment where those in the room did not have to survive. Some of the children I have worked with have spent their whole lives separated from their homelands, families, and communities, others had fled with their families, many had needed to grow up far faster than they should have. In these small experiences of the present moment, these children could be children. They could play and explore and imagine because it was safe to do so.

One young girl, Maya, who I worked with regularly, was eleven years old when we met. She was diagnosed with brittle bone disease at the age of one and in a wheelchair from age six. She is a remarkably joyful and resilient girl with a real sense of playfulness in her eyes. Maya was the resident artist at the community center where I worked, always creating, experimenting, and exploring. Her expressions of creativity were not about survival. It was where she had control and was free to do what felt right, or interesting, or exciting for her. We drew on this natural curiosity and creativity in our sessions. I observed so much joy when we practiced TCTSY together. Here we were not working at the level of survival either. The body became whole in some sense; it became a place to live and navigate, perhaps even to explore. And most beautifully for me as a facilitator, our bodies became places where we came together. Without the ability to stand, Maya played with how chairs could support her to create shapes and movements. We would work together to arrange a chair for her to hold as she folded forward or to rest her feet on when lifting her legs from the floor. We were connected and curious about each other's bodies without judgment, without any sense of the right or wrong way to do something. We simply asked the questions: How could we explore this shape? What possibilities does this form offer us? We might choose to experiment with a seated forward fold shape, perhaps extending our legs or crossing them and then maybe moving our upper body forward. What we found was that we could take our hands toward our feet, or we could bring a chair in front of us to hold and experiment with what it felt like to move our bodies in relation to another object. We could also sit on a blanket here, to notice if this changed how far forward we folded, or if it impacted on sensations in our legs or back. We shared ideas in these moments together, and in doing so, we learned from each other all the myriad ways there are to live in a body. Maya never appeared limited by her physical condition, although moving about in a wheelchair and needing to be carried up stairs, she very much lived in her body. What I feel our sessions offered her, and us as a group, was a chance to explore other ways of living and being.

I owe much gratitude to Maya for sharing her joy for life and hopeful spirit with me during our time together. Each day as I arrived at the community center Maya would open the door, smiling brightly and asking "*Yoga bugün?*"—"Yoga today?" I asked her on a number of occasions what she enjoyed about yoga. I asked in English, in Turkish, with an Arabic translator, through gestures and body language, and each time she shrugged. It seemed to me that it was beyond language, this thing that resonated with her when we practiced and moved together. Perhaps it was a moment when she was free to be herself, perhaps an opportunity to not have to worry about her brother or mother. Perhaps she felt seen or heard in this space together. I do not know, but language could not capture it. It was felt.

We interact with the world based on our felt sense of being in it— the contact of our feet with the ground as we walk, the sensation of hunger or thirst, experiences of temperature and pain. In TCTSY we are working with a present-moment experience centered on the body—centered on interoception, the awareness of how our body feels on the inside. Our interoceptive capacity dictates how we navigate our world, how we have our needs met, even how we respond to feelings and emotions. Interoceptive theory tells us that sensations come first, followed by an assessment of them: What are they communicating to us? From there we can take action based on the sensations we may notice. This is how we work with TCTSY, perhaps noticing sensations and then choosing how we respond to those sensations.

Offering TCTSY with children has been an experience of experimentation and exploration for me. I have found that naming sensations, and asking the children if they notice any particular sensations, has been helpful to identify and explore interoception. Unlike with my adult clients where the concept of sensations has often been clearer, children seemed to seek more information, more guidance. I found that once that framework was built, however, the children became curious to see what they noticed as they moved and breathed, how it felt to inhabit these living and breathing bodies.

We do not always work with the breath with TCTSY. For some survivors, the breath is not safe or accessible. The breath can be triggering for some, perhaps many, survivors of trauma. Some survivors' experiences may have involved being unable to breathe, struggling to catch their breath. Others may have lived for many years in a state of hyperarousal, in their stress response state. In this state breathing is often faster and shallower, and some survivors may be stuck here. Making a request or offering an invitation to "take a deep breath" can therefore feel either impossible or terrifying because they had survived by remaining hypervigilant and ready for fight or flight. I feel it is important to acknowledge that this is a protective and adaptive response that has served many of my clients incredibly well, keeping them alive. I ask my clients directly about their experience of their breath because they know if and how it serves them. They are the experts of their experience. For some survivors their breath is safe, an anchor from which to observe and feel some movement in their body. For others it is inaccessible or triggering. I am mindful of the spectrum of relationships with our breath in my work. While exploring movement and yoga with children, my experience has been that experimenting with tools such as pinwheels or feathers offers ways for them to see their breath and in this seeing to realize the impact, the agency, they may have on their environment and their world.

Working with Hassan was a joy for me as a facilitator as I watched this open and engaged young boy discover noticing and using his breath as a tool. Hassan was eight years old when we worked together; he had fled Syria with his family when he was four. He is bigender and living with cerebral palsy. When he first arrived at the community center he was unable to walk. Through regular physiotherapy he gained the ability to stand and walk aided with a frame. This new mobility brought him a genuine experience of freedom. He was very much part of the community, naturally out-going and seeking connections and opportunities to play. Hassan was also nonverbal, which meant that working with the body was a natural way to engage and connect for him. We used our cards and as many visual tools and resources as we could find. Hassan actively chose the forms he wanted to practice in our sessions. He knew how he wanted to practice and made choices to meet his needs and the needs and experiences of his body.

Hassan took to breath work with such curiosity and openness. The pinwheels were a favorite starting point for the breath. The colors and the movement brought giggles and excitement. How curious to see something spin without touching it. Then came some awareness that this breath moved in and out of our body and in this movement created a natural flow through our chest and stomach rising and falling. Belly breathing, as it is sometimes called, with our hands placed on our body was one of Hassan's favorites, and he often chose this form from the cards. I regularly observed him with his hands placed on his body, noticing the movement of his breath in his chest and stomach. Without language, we built a relation-ship with our bodies and our breath that, for me, opened my eyes to the many possibilities of the practice. Where connection and relationships are the key to healing from trauma, working nonverbally offers us a chance to build these connections across cultures and languages, across abilities and across ages.

What I was privileged to bear witness to in this work was a group of children who had thrived in their adversity and who, when given the chance to explore their bodies and their breath, fully inhabited them. These children knew how to live in their bodies, how to move without causing pain or injury. While their physical disabilities dictated how they moved around outside our sessions together, in a wheelchair or with the aid of a walking frame, in the sessions as we sat on the ground together, moved and breathed, twisted and folded our bodies, each one of them was whole. There did not appear to be a dichotomy between able-bodied and disabled; there was simply difference and diversity. Our differences were welcomed by the group as we supported each other and looked curiously at the shapes we inhabited and how we could change or adapt them to meet each of our needs.

The power of this program for me was in the group. In my social work career, I have specialized in group work because I believe that something transformative happens when we come together. When we bring people together for some shared means, in our case to explore movement based on our present-moment experience, a sense of community and belonging arises. We build connections and relationships, which are, after all, the heart of healing from trauma. The beauty of TCTSY in a group context with children living with a range of physical disabilities was the possibility to explore difference—different bodies, different abilities, different choices. To use curiosity, provide support, both physically as well as emotionally, and to move and breathe in rhythm with each other. All nonverbally. All bodily. All together.

Flowing with Chaos

Including Choice in Zen Buddhist Practice

Eric Daishin McCabe

The torch of chaos and doubt—this is what the sage steers by.

—CHUANG TZU[1]

The question was a simple one: "Would you prefer to practice today with the lights on or off?" I was within the initial five minutes of my first trauma-sensitive yoga class, which was held in a conference room with fluorescent lighting. It was a fair question from our instructor. But I was still lost in the anxiety of the new experience and in the idea that if I attended a yoga class such as this, then I was admitting the trauma by just being present, without saying a word. The instructor quietly asked again if we preferred the lights on or off. I had resolved to say nothing—this was my modus operandi. I looked to the girl to my left and then to the girl on my right; I knew that I would wait for one of them to make the decision. The question, as simple as it was, seemed overwhelming to me, and I honestly didn't feel as if I had a right to make any choice. I stayed quiet and the other girls opted to have the lights dimmed. I was pleased; the lights were too harsh and I recognized that for myself but I would have never voiced this nor made the decision unilaterally.

—YOGA STUDENT

WHAT FOLLOWS IS BY NO means the perspective of a trauma expert or of a Zen master, but of someone attempting to better understand trauma dynamics and learn more ways to apply practices found within yogic and Buddhist teachings. I have failed multiple times in this endeavor, yet I do everything I can to get back up again and again, keep my beginner's mind, and continue to learn from my mistakes.

All of my yoga and Buddhist teachers, as well as my blood family, have been instrumental in raising me up physically, psychologically, socially, and spiritually. For them and the way they have nurtured me I am grateful and forever indebted. While I can go into some depth about how I have benefited from their presence in my life, the purpose of this chapter is different. For this reason, I am hesitant to share my story. I sincerely wish no disrespect to anyone.

It is my hope that this writing will be a cause for reflection especially by teachers of Zen who are interested in or already offering the dharma to trauma survivors. Zen teachings can be incredibly powerful, and because the dharma can both heal and hurt depending on how it is applied and how it is received, it is vital that teachers who have vowed to save all sentient beings think deeply about whether their approaches are really beneficial for those with post-traumatic stress disorder (PTSD) or early childhood trauma. As a student of yoga, mindfulness, and Zen Buddhism for twenty-five years, I have witnessed and been a part of how unknowingly insensitive teachers, including myself, can be to trauma survivors, even while having the best of intentions to alleviate suffering. Here I share my own experiences, within my family of origin, within Zen communities, and with teaching Trauma Center Trauma-Sensitive Yoga (TCTSY) in a clinical setting. The investigation of my own story has helped me connect on a deeper level with and develop greater compassion for those I serve. My aim in this chapter, while not ignoring how deeply positive Zen has been to my life, is to shed light on the limitations of Zen philosophy and practices for attending to survivors, as well as ways in which TCTSY has helped hone how I offer Zen and facilitate yoga for those with mental health issues.

Anxiety has been a constant companion; my biggest fear is losing control. Externally, in my role as an instructor, this looks like students thinking differently from me, or of leaving the room without explanation. What this feels like internally is a racing heart, tightening abdomen, and a sense of panic and/or disconnection from my students and environment. I feel shame, self-doubt, and incompetence. Verbally (or within my own mind) I tell people what they "should" be doing or thinking.

Wanting order and control over myself and others, I reluctantly admit, has been a part of the fabric of my being ever since I can remember. Until studying trauma theory, I largely dismissed my childhood experiences of physical and verbal abuse and the witnessing of regular verbal altercations between my caregivers because, on a spectrum, it was not as extreme as other stories I had heard. I also felt sheltered from abuse that happened not only to immediate family but across familial generations. While I have had a lot of very positive and nurturing experiences in my family as well, I now realize the importance of bringing my shadow side more clearly into conscious awareness, for it is just as much a part of me—perhaps even influences me when I'm not fully present—as is my lighter side.

I also realize how easy it is for me to use the practice of dharma to justify ignoring my dark side with spiritual bypassing. In other words, feeling peace and happiness as a result of practicing meditation does not mean I have conquered the negative parts of me or that they no longer exist. That part of me will always be in me. Contrary to my previous beliefs, ignoring this dark side is inviting it to express itself without my attention. This is dangerous because then it comes out in ways that are harmful to me and others. Therefore, acknowledging my darkness as I do here is not a plea for sympathy but helps me be real, especially with survivors.

Alcohol and marijuana use, as well as obsession with pornography between the ages of fourteen and twenty-two, were part of a constellation of symptoms that may well be the result of the forms of abuse that I witnessed in my own life. It's hard for me to make a direct correlation, but when I think about the negative aspects of

my home life in the light of trauma theory, it makes the most sense
to me.

These obsessions strangely helped me feel more balanced and
whole, at least for a time. But then there would inevitably be a shift
out of balance, and into accompanying feelings of shame. The initial release from pain brought enough relief, and with nothing else
to replace these behaviors, it was enough to create and maintain a
habit. It's thanks to these early experiences that I am able to connect on some level with many clients. My symptoms, I believe, were
exacerbated by the hyper-competitive world of swimming that I had
been a part of during those years, and they greatly abated once I
met my Buddhist teacher and began to practice meditation and
study the dharma at the age of twenty.

My perceived need to excel academically and athletically contributed to experiences of anxiety beyond, perhaps, what could be
considered constructive. The idea of having agency over myself,
having the ability to choose what I want, was largely foreign to me
until years into my adulthood. Today I am often challenged when
offered genuine choices. I disbelieve what I'm presented with, and
I prefer others to make choices for me.

As I began to realize that I could make choices that would not
necessarily please family, there was backlash. As a child I wasn't
given the opportunity to choose which clothes to wear. If I was wearing something that did not meet my mother's standards she would
insist that I change. Perhaps this seems like an insignificant rule,
but looking more closely, it is no small thing, for it mirrored many
other experiences where I had no choice or agency. In college, for
instance, when I had to choose a major and decided on religion, I
think the only reason my parents allowed it was that I majored in
biology as well. My parents scorned the academic study of religion
because they believed it would not make me more economically
viable. Each of my parents had their own ideas about religion. At
the time, I perceived them as disconnected from, and either unin-
terested or fearful about, what I was learning. My parents hated
that I was not subscribing to their ideas about success and what

it means to become an adult. I truly believe they meant well. The fact that I chose to study religion felt like a big deal to me. In hindsight my parents' reluctant support, living away from home, and having excellent guidance from my professors all encouraged me in making this decision.

In college I came to Zen through an existential crisis brought on by the study of religion, lack of helpful social support, marijuana and alcohol abuse, and a broken heart. As I had been studying religion, it began to dawn on me that the meanings I had ascribed to God were flimsy at best. I believed one thing but acted in ways that were contrary to those beliefs. I didn't fully comprehend the idea I had learned in the Catholic church, for example, that I am unconditionally loved by God, though that was what I had been taught. I had not translated the teaching well into practice. I had a considerable amount of self-loathing. Why else would I feel the need to use?

Part of my crisis also came from a new understanding in college of my place in the social fabric of the world and of US society. I began to see that life isn't all about me but that there is a wider world that I am responsible for. I learned that my ancestors were liable for the genocide of Native peoples and for the slavery of Africans, justified by the supposed superiority of Christian and Eurocentric beliefs. Further I learned that I am a beneficiary of policies that disproportionately benefit white people over people of color. These policies—which enable white people, for example, access to better housing and education—have their basis in unchecked racist attitudes but remain disguised in a system based on meritocracy. Even though I work to not perpetuate racism, I am part of and support—even on an unconscious level—a system that rewards me for being white. Learning this, there was no way I could put the "jack back in the box." I could no longer see the world in the glorified way my pre-college days had presented it to me.

The contradictions I met within myself regarding my relationship with God and my place in the larger society were not reconcil-
able. I began to question God's existence, and as a result my own
purpose in life. If God did not exist, then why am I here? If there
is no God that cares about me personally, then where does my existence come from, and why should I care what I do?

During this transformative period, I found my Zen teacher. I wasn't
looking for Zen. In a sense, Zen found me. In one of my religion
classes we watched a demonstration of zazen, or sitting meditation.
What I remembered most about that video was that the teacher
did not mention a thing about God, that he appeared totally at
peace, and that his words matched his actions. I wanted to learn
more. Shortly after that video, without looking for it, I happened to
notice that another teacher was regularly offering Zen meditation
on campus, and she had been for the past three years. I had never
known about it until that moment. I decided to meet her.

Simply sitting next to her in stillness and silence I felt peace. She
too didn't talk about God, and she encouraged me to more deeply
explore the questions I had about life purpose, calling it my koan.
A koan is a conundrum that cannot be adequately solved by linear-
sequential thinking. Practitioners of Zen, rather, "sit" with the koan
like a hen sitting on an egg, not knowing what the results will be. This
kind of sitting helps one connect more fully with the mystery at the
foundation of life. This teacher, who later became my root teacher,
taught me that it was okay to "not know" and to sit with this "not knowing" with openness and curiosity. After my first meeting with her I felt
better than I'd ever felt without having smoked marijuana or binged
on alcohol. I knew that this was a path I needed to stick with, and while
I have not missed a day of Zen meditation since that first day meeting
my teacher, I had no idea then that I would become a Zen priest.

My parents did not know what to make of me as I was waking up
to the impermanence and fragility of life on this planet for humans

and all species. I saw destruction and death happening at an unprecedented rate all around me, and it's as though I was being encouraged to disregard it or numb myself to it and carry on with business as usual. When I eventually chose to live in a Zen temple, my father, bless him, told me to get checked for schizophrenia. He must have been terribly worried about me. My mother was so angry that she threatened to disown me. They said these things, I'm convinced, because they did not have the language to process what they were feeling or the tools for adequate self-reflection. I have no feelings of resentment toward them for their reactions. To the contrary, their disapproval was exactly the resistance I needed at the time to carry my plans forward. I needed to make a decision that was clearly mine, not something handed to me.

Following several years of training in the Zen center, and of my parents showing concern for my mental health, I suggested we go to a therapist together and hear a professional's opinion. This turned to my favor when the therapist suggested to my parents that they needed to let go of me, that I was an adult and could figure things out for myself. While this move appeared to be a win, I still felt a deep ache in the pit of my stomach. There was a part of me that longed for remaining in the kind of unhealthy pattern I had had with my parents.

Ironically, the path I chose to commit myself to, Zen Buddhism, does not emphasize making choices as a practice. Rather, the emphasis is on fully embodying the forms that have been passed down through the generations and expressing one's life force through those forms. This is a beautiful practice, but it may have serious repercussions for those with trauma. In many of the meditation centers I attended in Japan, for example, I was expected to sit in either full or half lotus posture when meditating, and in seiza (with feet folded under my sit bones) during other activities, totally ignoring knee pain or indications that my body was giving me to move. This is, consequently, one of the reasons I took up yoga. Yoga helped me loosen my body up so that I could sit in those postures. But in Japanese and some American Zen temples I always felt self-conscious about practicing yoga, and I would do it as secretly as possible. Yogic practices were seen by some teachers as incompatible with Zen.

Today I see this insistence on conforming to a physical form as one example of a problematic teaching when it comes to working with trauma survivors: When teachers tell students what to do with their body, they risk triggering past memories of when choice was taken away. The student may then be inadvertently pulled into the past, going the opposite direction of what was intended by the teacher. Instead of listening to one's body, a student may perceive this instruction as an expectation to demonstrate loyalty to the wisdom of a teacher, thereby reaffirming a distrust of the signals coming from their own physical body.

When I was first introduced to meditation practice, my Zen teacher told me what to do with my body and thoughts. She taught how to comport my legs, back, arms, neck, and head while sitting still and in silence. The meditation room at the campus's chapel is where meditation was held. It was a large and spacious room with a very high ceiling. Upon entering, I saw my teacher leaned over as she was setting out black zafus in a circular pattern and massaging the cushions so they were puffy. My teacher was very welcoming, and I felt her warm smile.

She instructed me to join my palms together and bow to the cushion I was to sit on, to turn clockwise and then bow to the others in the circle. Sitting upon the cushion, I was directed to sit on the front third, helping to tilt my pelvis forward, so that my knees would be lower than my abdomen. As far as my torso was concerned she instructed by saying, "Ears, shoulders, and hips in one plane, nose and navel in one line, neither leaning left nor right, forward nor backward. Eyes are left half open looking downward and with a soft gaze. Lift the nape of the neck. Count your breaths from one to ten and back to one. When thoughts come into your mind, drop them, returning to the breath." At the end of the meditation period, marked by the sound of a bell, all participants brought their palms together and bowed once again in unison, turned to face their cushions, puffed them up, and then stood and proceeded to do walking meditation in unison.

As a beginner, I appreciated simply learning about how to use my body from someone who had more experience than me with meditation. Simply following someone else's instructions brought great benefit. I found myself immediately more focused just by aligning my back properly. In sitting still, I felt at peace inside. I never knew that kind of peace or that it was so accessible to me. Had I not had the instruction to sit still and had it modeled exquisitely, I don't think I would have been able to do it.

After graduating college I did a stint teaching English in Japan for one year then returned to the United States to begin a graduate program in religion. Shortly into the program I became disillusioned about the academic study of religion. Here I was in my early twenties, and it struck me as quite odd that I could think deeply about religious subjects but have little ability to cook for myself or take care of my basic needs. This felt unbalanced and embarrassing. I opted to drop out of graduate school and become an emergency substitute teacher. I didn't need a teaching certificate to do this, and it would get my feet wet in the real world. No doubt it was challenging to work with children of all ages as a substitute, but I at least felt like I was connecting with people in real life where they were, as opposed to sitting at a desk and writing philosophical papers that had no basis in anything that seemed relevant to me—at least at that time.

I eventually landed back home with my parents where I found full-time work as a fifth-grade teacher in a Catholic school. Having had little experience teaching fifth graders, and being somewhat naïve about the politics in schools, I found myself in over my head, unable to "control" the class. After five months of struggle I was asked to resign, and I did so reluctantly.

Now I was without work, having failed at getting a graduate degree, and a choice opened up for me. What would I do in this new space? I could go back to school to get a teacher's certification with the expectation that I could be hired elsewhere, or I could train with the Zen teacher who initially taught me Zen meditation. I had kept in touch with her and attended a few of her retreats after graduating college. I knew she was trying to run a Zen center and, at that time, had no one in residence.

Did I want to get a degree in order to return to a similar situation only a little better prepared? Or could I really learn what this meditation practice that had so profoundly affected me was about? Could I really put more effort into aligning my values with the reality of my life, something I felt was glaringly absent? I saw the opportunity to learn from a master as quite rare. Would this opportunity ever present itself again? Having no job or family to take care of became a gift because it allowed me to, so to speak, take the next step off the top of a 100-foot pole. I had no idea at the time where this would lead, that I would become a priest, meet several other great masters, return to Japan, and basically live a temple-centered life for the next fifteen years.

My life for those years was marked by early morning rising to sit in meditation, chanting sutras, cooking, cleaning, gardening, doing all the activities needed to run a temple, and listening to instruction and feedback from my teacher with regards to many of the aspects of my life. I was the treasurer, assistant to my teacher, board member, and eventually took on teaching roles. My life, for the most part, felt fairly balanced between physical labor and mental exercise. Every day I was physically active, using my arms and legs to wipe down floors and chop cabbage or other vegetables. I found stillness in retreats that were anywhere from one day to seven days in length—focusing primarily on sitting meditation. I felt integrated into the wider community, offering meditation to college students in several local colleges, being a guest teacher, being a part of interfaith gatherings, working as an aide at a nursing home, and teaching meditation at the drug and alcohol rehab. I had found a sense of meaning that went beyond the narrow ideas I had held about God and was able to be deeply critical of the norms and expectations of a white man in our society.

I had no idea then that being told what to do with my legs, arms, and back could actually be triggering for some people. Nor did it ever occur to me that my experience of my body could actually be different from someone who I thought had more experience with theirs. On an unconscious level I assumed that a teacher could know my body better than I could know my own. I was sold on Zen, reluctant to question guidance from a teacher, including the instruction to subdue one's wish to choose.

This practice of refraining from choice is centuries old and has been memorialized and glorified in the ancient Zen poem entitled "Faith in Mind." This poem is recited frequently at many Zen centers in the United States. The very first two lines convey a central message of training toward the goal of Enlightenment: "The Great Way is not difficult, just don't pick and choose. If you cut off all likes and dislikes, everything is clear like space."[2] In other words, the path to Enlightenment lies in one's ability to subdue one's personal choices and open up to what the Universe is presenting in the moment. This sometimes translated into doing what those more experienced and senior than you ask. The hierarchy built into many Zen communities, while meant to preserve peace and order, has the downside of creating students uncritical of those in a higher rank. In this hierarchy, advanced students are able to simply do what is asked of them by the teacher without question or hesitation. The reasoning behind this is the dissolution of ego. The price for group harmony is letting go of one's personal preferences. The positive aspect of this practice is having a sense of place and of group unity, something that is often lacking in cultures like the United States', which prides itself on individual expression.

However, these instructions may be devastating for anyone in recovery from trauma. They can mirror an abusive dynamic that many trauma survivors experienced within their family or in their relationship with an abusive person. Zen culture in many ways mirrored an abusive dynamic found in my own family. For example, any food that was offered to the community as alms had to be received and consumed. There is the teaching that a "monk's mouth is like an oven." An oven cooks whatever is put into it without discrimination. While this is a profound teaching about growing one's capacity to let go of preference, thereby aligning oneself with Enlightenment, another outcome is ignoring the Buddha wisdom that is manifesting in one's own body here and now. Being full yet feeling pressure to eat from senior students or teachers is ignoring the wisdom of the Buddha in one's own body. Judith Herman writes, "The first principle of recovery is the empowerment of the survivor. She must be the author and arbiter of her own recovery."[3] Not allowing someone the opportunity to make a choice, to discern for themselves what to eat and what not to eat, *is* taking power away from them. The sense of agency in that person atrophies.

Another place where subduing choice became a problem for me was with regards to struggles with loneliness and lack of intimacy connected to, I suspect, pornography use as an adolescent. Twenty years of celibacy, though I wasn't conscious of it at the time, was my way of working through porn addiction. Pornography had, I believe, numbed me to or robbed me of the need for real intimacy. The practice of celibacy became a powerful antidote for restoring my vitality, allowing me to feel what was real within me, as opposed to being sideswiped again and again by erotic images. Thanks in part to maintaining a celibate lifestyle, I had deep breakthroughs where I could really see that I am more than my body or mind, that I am this universe. There were times I felt deep intimacy with all living things.

Ironically, with the restoration of my vitality came an even stronger need to really connect with another human being, and for me that meant being in a committed monogamous relationship.

Feelings of loneliness grew stronger until I realized that I could no longer maintain the practice as I had understood it. I had great anxiety in totally owning up to my feelings because I didn't know how they would be received by others in my community and was not clear about the consequences. Once I did share my feelings, I realized the need to transition out of the Zen center.

Deep feelings of loss and shame accompanied me in this transition not because of my choice to end the practice of celibacy or to leave the Zen center, but because of the very act of choosing what was real. I believe this conscious choice triggered bodily memories of past events where I was shamed for choosing what felt real. Perhaps I was afraid to choose what was real for me in the long run because that meant I would need to change the familiarity of my then-present experience, as well as need to deal with my past. I held off on really listening to what my body-mind was communicating to me for as long as I physically and psychologically could. Another way to put it is that the antidote—celibacy—that helped immensely for a certain time period, especially as I was clarifying what was real and working through addiction, had to be reevaluated because of the new information I was receiving from my own body. I had to take seriously what my own body was communicating to me, and that meant I needed to make a conscious choice of how I was to proceed. The Zen teaching of "just don't pick and choose," while effective under certain conditions, with regard to the issue of intimacy became a way of bypassing or ignoring my own physical and emotional needs.

I did not begin to reflect on how the way I was trained could do more harm for trauma survivors until I began teaching meditation and yoga at an in-patient drug and alcohol rehab, located just thirty minutes' drive from the Zen temple where I was residing. In 2010 a counselor from the rehab invited me to offer Zen meditation for those in recovery. I had an intuitive sense that these were my people. I knew addiction on some level. I'd witnessed it in myself and family. I knew that meditation was a way to deal with addiction, and I was eager to share the practice, thinking others in recovery would also benefit in similar ways to me.

For me, meditation was a gateway to self-acceptance. I could more willingly open up to the various parts of myself that I was ashamed of. Prior to knowing about meditation, I felt the need to put on a facade of happiness and wherewithal. Meditation, along with compassionate instruction from teachers, helped me see and embrace my dark side—that I don't have my act together, that I have faults, and that I can never know fully who I am. Whether I want it or not, this body-mind I have come to identify with is not all that I am. Furthermore, mini "Enlightenment" experiences after or during meditation, where I felt profoundly in sync with the natural world, helped me let go of the need to seek special experiences through marijuana. My teachers discouraged seeking after such experiences, imploring me to return to the reality that is right before me. Only here and now can Enlightenment be found. Let go of the past.

These realizations and teachings are potentially liberating for anyone in recovery. Lack of self-acceptance, denial of one's dark sides, overidentification with one's body-mind, and desperately seeking connection to something or someone greater than oneself are hallmarks of addiction and things that every one of us struggles with on some level. If meditation could address these in me, certainly it could be of great benefit to others as well.

The campus of the rehab was seated among rolling mountains, in a well wooded and sheltered area. There were several buildings including dormitories separating men and women, a cafeteria, administrative buildings, and common rooms for various activities, including my class. There would usually be fifteen to twenty clients in my group (and once I introduced yoga I had more than forty);

however, there were also several times when I had only a few attend, or even no one, especially when I first began teaching.

In my early experiences at the rehab, I taught the way I had been taught, and I mistakenly assumed my clients lacked self-discipline. I had clients conforming to the posture that I had been taught (with the exception of requesting full or half lotus), sitting in silence, and asking that they remain still for the entire period of a meditation, which usually lasted five to ten minutes. Within this style, my anxiety level would begin as moderate, then either increase exponentially if I did not feel a sense of control over the external environment, or decrease if I felt that I was being given "proper" attention. Teaching Zen was not just about offering students techniques that could help them, but about me. I had an unconscious desire to be at the center of things. Not that I didn't care about the students, but I was not adequately imagining myself in their shoes, nor did I fully understand the role that the deeper layers of trauma were playing for them or me.

A turning point occurred for me when a colleague introduced me to Gabor Maté's book *In the Realm of Hungry Ghosts*.[4] Upon reading, I was struck by the connection Maté drew between addiction and trauma. Most people with opioid addiction issues had some early childhood trauma such as physical abuse, sexual abuse, or neglect, according to Maté. It dawned on me that I needed much deeper compassion for my clients, and that most forms of discipline coming from me were totally inappropriate in such a setting. Discipline may be interpreted from the perspective of the survivor as another form of abuse. From the perspective of the "teacher" the idea may be that discipline will prevent or end disruptive behavior. But trauma survivors often experience the world as an unsafe place, and people as not worthy of trust. Most forms of discipline without a deeper understanding of the underlying unprocessed pain are misguided because, rather than ending bad behavior, they generate more mistrust and solidify the idea that the world is unsafe.

I began to recognize that those in recovery are doing everything they can to get rid of their pain, stored in their bodies over the years. Drugs are, for them, a way to alleviate that pain. They were doing what they knew to feel better, even if it was for short-term alleviation. In my experience with marijuana I felt the freedom to be myself, to think the way that I wanted, and to speak my mind, without feeling cut off. I was also able to better feel my emotions. It was (and in many ways still is) extraordinarily painful for me to keep my true feelings to myself. On an unconscious level I suppress how I feel. I only come to know I'm suppressing when I have the presence of mind to begin to look at my own mind. I may come to see that I have a strong feeling that something is not right. Anger is often the surface emotion in this case. Underlying this anger are usually grief and feelings of not belonging. Drugs, particularly my brief experiments with LSD and psilocybin, helped me get in touch with that grief, to be with it, to allow it, to accept it on some level.

My perception of the rehab clients changed from drug abusers lacking self-discipline to survivors. With this paradigm shift came a physical/psychological opening in my heart-center. While I was teaching, tightness in my abdomen and the emotion of fear slowly transformed to spaciousness and a feeling of compassion.

I recognized as fiction the notion that addiction is caused by taking drugs. This "just say no" idea reveals a society-wide ignorance regarding both the way the brain develops and the importance of early childhood attachment. "Just say no" comes from the assumption that someone with addiction is in a place to make a choice. It implies that one has had plenty of practice making choices, but it ignores the reality that most survivors were denied choice.

I taught at the rehab once a week for roughly three years, between 2010 and 2013. Even without having any formal training in trauma dynamics, once my perception of the clients changed, I received consistent positive feedback from the literally hundreds of clients I had served during that time. What was most palpably different for me was a feeling of compassion. These were folks who were hurt as children and never received adequate or appropriate care at those times. I began to imagine them as wounded. Discipline was not an appropriate response to their disheveled appearance and disorganized thoughts.

I encouraged clients to sit either on the floor or in chairs. Sitting in a chair is generally frowned upon in Zen temples, and for the most part forbidden in Japanese Zen temples. One reason for this is that sitting on a chair places one in a physically higher position than a teacher, who presumably would be sitting on the floor (or perhaps a raised platform). While most Zen centers in the United States accommodate for chairs, still there is an unspoken sense of the inferiority of that position for meditation, as well as an unwritten agreement of it being disrespectful toward the teacher. I can't emphasize enough how ingrained this thinking is among Zen practitioners, and even among society at large, particularly among those who have never tried to mediate. We associate "proper" meditation to sitting cross-legged on the floor whether we've meditated or not. This is a major barrier for most beginners, especially those intimidated by the prospects of having to conform their legs to a variation of lotus.

After instructions to sit either on the floor or in a chair, I'd proceed to introduce myself—not neglecting to share that I too have struggles with addiction, and that meditation and yoga have helped me alleviate the pain in my life. I noticed that until I self-disclosed, clients were less open to listening to me. But once I became more authentic in sharing my experience, I could feel a lightening in the room. People's bodies, I could see, physically softened. It was then that I would begin meditation instruction.

I would vary the direction in which we sat. Sometimes we would face inward, in a circle; other times we would face outward toward the wall. The benefit to facing the wall was that the clients did not feel like they were being watched all the time.

Many approached me afterward saying that not only did they feel better, but this meditation should be offered every day. People often commented that the tone of my voice was soothing and helped them to settle. They even asked me to record myself so

that they could listen to my voice. I took these as signals that I was
moving in the right direction.

After about six months of my offering Zen meditation, the counselor
who had been my liaison asked if I would also teach yoga to his clients. I said I would, but under the condition that I get formally certified to do so. Because of the rigors of Zen practice, I always found
yoga an important accompaniment to meditation. It was not a big
stretch for me to expand my offering, and I was lucky enough to have
the support of my Zen community to do the training, as well as the
patience of the rehab to wait six months for me to begin.

Once I began teaching, I found I enjoyed offering yoga to the
clients because of how much positive feedback I was receiving.
When one of my Zen colleagues learned I had been teaching yoga
at the rehab, she gave me a copy of David Emerson's book *Overcoming Trauma through Yoga.*[5] I have to admit that I did not immediately
find the book remarkable, nor did I read through it thoroughly,
and because of the relative success I was feeling from what I was
doing, it sat on my shelf for about four years.

In 2013 I transitioned from the Zen center where I had been
training for fifteen years into a one-year chaplaincy training program at a hospital a couple of hours away. Because of my work
at the rehab, I chose to work on the Behavioral Health Unit so I
could better understand psychological disorders. I was a spiritual
counselor to more than a thousand patients that year, almost all
of whom had some form of addiction and underlying childhood
trauma. While I benefited greatly from this experience, learning
excellent counseling skills, what I missed most about the work
was teaching body awareness as I had done at the rehab through
meditation and yoga.

I found that most of my patients at the hospital were replaying old tapes in their heads, and my work as a chaplain was not to tell them what to think or believe but to help them uncover their own spiritual resources and facilitate access to them. Even though spiritual counseling was of some benefit, I became acutely aware of the importance of the grounding that takes place in both myself and others during the practice of yoga and meditation, especially because I felt its absence while in the role of chaplain.

At the end of that internship, I moved several hundred miles away to be with my wife-to-be. She had been working in domestic-violence prevention overseas for many years when we met at the Zen center where I'd been living. When I transitioned to my chaplaincy work our relationship commenced, and we decided to marry and to live with my in-laws for the year while she continued to work from home and I looked for meaningful work in a place that was totally new and unfamiliar to me.

I knew that I wanted to offer yoga in a behavioral health setting as a way of bringing together my experiences as a chaplain and as a yoga teacher working with addiction. I researched hospitals in the area that had inpatient behavioral health programs and asked those in charge if they were interested in having a yoga teacher for their patients. I also made connections with therapists, letting them know of my skillset. This outreach led to contracted work where I offered yoga for inpatient and outpatient mental health, as well as with an outpatient addiction treatment program. I also met a therapist who offered me space in his office to teach yoga on the condition that I do training in trauma-sensitive yoga. I was eager to learn specifically about trauma-sensitive yoga, and David Emerson happened to be offering a workshop to yoga teachers just a three-hour drive from where I was.

What I got from David's presence was much different from what I had initially read in his book. In a way, the book didn't make sense to me until I saw how he taught in person. The strong emphasis on *really* offering yoga students the opportunity to make choices within the context of a yoga class struck me. David would often pause after offering choice and reiterate the choices, and he seemed to check for a nonverbal sense that people really understood that they had the power to choose and that there was no stigma around that choosing. In contrast, at the Zen and yoga centers I practiced at where choice was offered, I often felt or perceived that there was a better choice, and that I needed to work on "improving" my choices so they aligned with an aim of perfection. As I practiced making choices during the course of the training, I could feel a sense of space and calm open in my head and around my heart. Moreover, I began to offer choice to clients I had been working with both privately and at the hospital.

Before meeting David, I had been working with a student (whom I'll refer to as Jack to protect his identity) from Beijing who was studying electrical engineering at the local university. He was referred to me by a therapist with the suggestion to teach him mindfulness practices for anxiety.

Jack was in his late twenties, had been in the United States studying for seven years, expressed feeling isolated from family, and had concerns about his weight. His anxiety was triggered by the recent ending of a romantic relationship. He was also preparing to graduate and leave for further schooling in California. During the course of our conversations I learned that he had been placed in a boarding school at six years of age and scolded by his parents that he was spoiled. Furthermore, in opposition to his father, he desired to become something other than an electrical engineer.

I had been giving Jack personal instruction in mindfulness techniques, teaching him ways to comport his body and mind and do walking meditation, all practices that I had learned from my teachers. I also prescribed these practices for him to do when anxiety was strong.

After completing the short seminar with David Emerson, I began to take a different approach with Jack. I stopped prescribing meditation, and I began offering choices. In my notes I wrote:

> I taught Jack after returning from the TCTSY workshop. I was able to see immediate results when I put TCTSY into practice—particularly in regards to offering Jack choices as to where to put his attention in meditation.
>
> At the start of the class he began to talk about an issue that came up with his therapist. Practicing TCTSY, I gave him the choice to continue talking about that issue or to do yoga. He requested to do meditation.
>
> Within meditation he brought up some of the difficulties he has in doing meditation on his own. I let go of the idea of trying to get him to see the importance of meditating regularly because, just the thought of that is entering into a future-oriented practice. I instead gave Jack a few choices of where to put his attention when his mind was full of thoughts—mainly on the thumbs, limbs and/or spine. Jack also had questions about how to use his eyes, and, again, I gave him options of where to put his gaze.
>
> He immediately put my suggestions into practice and was eager to continue meditating.
>
> I gave him the bell to ring so that he was in charge of deciding how long to sit for. My intention was to empower him, and it involved me letting go of my own agenda and trusting that he would know when and how to end it.
>
> Because of the issue with his father, I now understand the importance of allowing him choices.

I cannot overstate the shift I felt within my own body-mind in the process of working with Jack from a trauma-sensitive perspective. I had evolved from a place of telling Jack how to do practice in order to relieve anxiety to one of giving him choices. In offering him choices I was giving him the opportunity to cultivate a sense of agency. He had the chance to see the options available to him and then choose what to do. This shift in my own style of teaching precipitated feelings of spaciousness and freedom, as well as an acceptance of the natural anxiety that comes with letting go of trying to control other people. In Jack, I noticed stillness and curiosity. I had facilitated a sense of agency in him by offering choices.

At the hospital where I taught yoga classes to mental health patients, the way I taught began to shift, too. Here is a typical class on the inpatient Behavioral Health Unit after completing certification in TCTSY:

> I use my black wrist band to enter into a locked-down space. Hanging from one shoulder is my blue duffle bag full of eight yoga mats. The weight of the bag presses down on my shoulders, keeping me grounded. I am dressed in blue jeans and a plain shirt so that I don't draw unnecessary attention to myself. I see patients identified by their green hospital-issued pants and shirts. Some are pacing the halls. Others are sitting at tables staring, playing cards, or watching TV. I meet with the activities coordinator, and she helps me set up a side room by moving tables and chairs to one side, and then helping recruit patients who would like to do yoga.
>
> I greet everyone that's present with a warm and subtle smile and let them know that I'll be offering Trauma-Sensitive Yoga and that they are welcome to join. Then I move from patient to patient personally introducing myself and inviting them to class. I let them know they don't have to stay for the whole thing. They can leave at any time. Some I've seen before; many I'm meeting for the first time.
>
> One patient has gotten several of the other patients excited about doing yoga, so I have a room of about nine patients plus myself. The walls of the room are glass so that patients and staff can see in and out. There are curtains

available to conceal the glass walls, and I ask the patients if they would prefer to have the curtains drawn or open.

The patients request to have the lights dim, taking agency over their environment. I ask them where they would like me to stand. Depending on the class, I sometimes give the patients a brief intro to TCTSY so they know what it's about; other times I drop the introduction, especially if I'm sensing no patience for explanations. I listen to the cues from my own body as to how to proceed.

I give the option to connect the movement of their arms with their breath, and we begin. Within the first couple of minutes one person gets up to leave, then another follows her. I thank them for coming in. A person who peers in from outside sees what's going on and comes in. I welcome her, pointing to an empty mat. I let people know that we all don't have to be doing the same thing, they can rest at any time, and they are always welcome to return if they decide to leave the room.

Five people are following my movements, one person is lying down, and another is doing what looks like karate. I roll with the chaos, letting go of trying to make everyone conform to my movements. Within fifteen minutes there is more coming and going in the room. I ask the students if there are any yoga forms they would like to do or parts of their body that they want to work on. Some are startled by the shift in power, and others run with it, eager to define the class. After more time, we shift to lying on our backs and then to resting. Coming out of resting I see noticeable changes in those who stayed for the whole class. Some report feeling a lessening of anxiety and express their gratitude; others just leave.

Thanks to my years of training in meditation and a deeper understanding of trauma and ways to implement choice in the context of a yoga class, I find myself much more comfortable with the chaos I experience on the inpatient Behavioral Health Unit. I don't feel the need to be in charge as strongly. At times, I notice how attached I am to the results, feeling bad when I think I've not made an impact. Then I remind myself that my practice is to let go of the outcome. While I notice in myself much less anxiety around teaching yoga for patients on a mental health unit, I am also aware of my own tendencies, even after all my training, to want to be in control. I also am aware of the importance of holding myself accountable for my past actions. My past informs me in the present, it connects me with my students, and it keeps me attentive to my dark side. Doing my utmost to flow with the chaos of the moment, my work is never complete.

"I Was Able to
Take Something Back"

Empowerment and Self-Trust after Sexual Violence

Rowan Silverberg

THE ROOTS OF MY INTEREST in embodied approaches to healing from sexual and gender-based violence extend deep into the ground of my childhood. Born in 1956, I spent the first four years of my life in rural northwestern Ohio. In my earliest memory, I am four years old. Standing on top of a woodpile near my family's home, I feel the freshness of the autumn air, the peace of the early morning. I see a horse across the road, head lowered as he quietly eats grass in an apple orchard. I feel so happy to be alive and excited about the possibility of a new day. This enduring, embodied sense of joy and vibrant enthusiasm has stayed with me over these many years, despite the challenges that have also marked my life.

I am an incest survivor. Throughout my girlhood and adolescence, I learned to suppress my truths and bury my emotions. It was a long struggle to emerge from this state of separation from my embodied experience and gradually regain the capacity to trust myself—to feel what I feel, know what I know, and speak from a place of connection to my own experience.

Much to my good fortune, I discovered yoga at the age of nine when the book *Yoga for Americans* practically fell off the school library shelf into my hands.[1] Although I had learned to become frozen and silent in order to cope with sexual abuse, through yoga I was able to connect to something inside me that was alive and true. As I worked with basic movement and breathing sequences presented in the book, I often felt a sense of grace and freedom that was paralleled only by the feeling of expansiveness and peace I felt in the natural world. I continued to practice on my own and eventually started to attend classes when I was in my late teens and early twenties. I trained in a variety of approaches to yoga (anusara, iyengar, ashtanga vinyasa, kripalu) and began teaching yoga in 1990. I taught community classes and offered sessions as part of my work in a primary care clinic.

In 2014 I discovered Trauma Center Trauma-Sensitive Yoga (TCTSY) and began working as a volunteer at a rape crisis center in the urban Midwestern US city in which I lived. I had a desire to serve as an ally to survivors of sexual violence; I was motivated by the vision of eventually integrating yoga into peer support groups at the rape crisis center. For a year I took calls on the twenty-four-hour crisis hotline and was a "face-to-face" advocate, which included accompanying survivors of sexual assault to hospital emergency rooms and police stations. Concurrently I enrolled in a training program at the Trauma Center in Brookline, Massachusetts, in order to become certified as a TCTSY facilitator.

Rosalita and Starr were two members of a TCTSY peer support group I co-facilitated at the rape crisis center during the first half of 2016. In this support group, a TCTSY practice (initially ten to fifteen minutes, gradually increasing to thirty to forty-five minutes) was integrated into ninety-minute sessions that met once weekly for twelve consecutive weeks. The group was offered to adult women survivors of sexual violence as an adjunct to clinical mental health treatment for PTSD.

Seven individuals participated in this particular twelve-week series, which was co-facilitated by a licensed psychotherapist employed by the rape crisis center. The group was present centered and focused on providing opportunities for survivors to enhance awareness of present-moment embodied experience, expand available coping strategies and decision-making skills, and diminish isolation and self-blame. Potential participants were either referred to the group by therapists who were employed by the rape crisis center or they were self-referred. Individuals who referred themselves learned about the group from the rape crisis center's website or through word of mouth. Since February 2016 groups have been offered consistently at two locations for clients of this agency.

In a doctoral dissertation study, I explored the narratives of seven members of the TCTSY peer support group.[2] This research focused on the story each participant told of her experiences in the group and the impact of those experiences in her life. Research data was collected at three open-ended interviews: initial interviews were conducted one to two months after the support group's conclusion; second interviews took place eight to nine months after the first interview; final interviews occurred approximately eighteen months after the second interview. All quotes in this essay were taken from Rosalita and Starr's original research data.

Rosalita

When Rosalita joined the peer support group, she was fifty years old. In her own words, she characterized herself as "empathetic, trustworthy, and quirky." Wondering what she meant by "quirky," I inquired about this. Rosalita replied by saying that she often has a unique viewpoint and characterized herself as having a childlike appreciation for wonder, particularly in relation to nature and animals.

Initially Rosalita was motivated to become a member of the group because she had struggled alone for over twenty years with the aftermath of sexual violence. From Rosalita's perspective, trauma had negatively affected her sense of identity and compromised her capacity for growth. Rosalita was hopeful that, over the course of the twelve-week group, she might begin to free herself from the limitations that the trauma of sexual violence had imposed on her.

In addition, she believed that participation might help her begin to cultivate greater peace in her life.

During our first interview in June 2016, Rosalita articulated her motivation for becoming part of this group.

> *It had been . . . so many years that I hadn't dealt with [the trauma] . . . I never went to therapy until now and I was willing to try anything that would help. Really anything, because I was so stuck, and I wanted to feel . . . more freedom. I felt stuck [in the sense that the trauma] defined me as a person. In my mind, yoga always meant being peaceful. And I thought, "Wow, wouldn't that feel nice, to feel peaceful?" That's how I interpreted it.*

The yoga portion of the initial support group session was ten to fifteen minutes long. During the first practice Rosalita experienced self-consciousness and self-judgment. Wondering if she was doing the practice correctly, Rosalita, like almost all the other participants, focused on exteroception, an externally defined perception of self, rather than interoception, an internally oriented perception of self and embodied experience. Reflecting on her first experience of the TCTSY practice, Rosalita recalled,

> *It was a definite progression . . . initially, you're almost hesitant . . . you feel uncomfortable with yourself; you're judging yourself: "Oh my gosh, what's everybody else doing? Am I doing it right?" . . . I remember the time where [you invited us to notice] our feet on the ground and . . . I got very emotional because I only wanted one foot on the ground. I didn't want the other foot on the ground.*

In one of our conversations, Rosalita reflected on her experience of not wanting to feel both feet on the ground during that first yoga practice.

> *At that time, I didn't want to be part of the world. Whenever I felt physically and emotionally uncomfortable, I would distance myself . . . I almost felt as if I wasn't on the ground, I was up there watching myself. So, if something happened that made me feel uncomfortable, I would block it out, and I would literally take myself to a different place.*

When I'm experiencing dissociation, I feel completely disconnected with earth. I feel more comfortable not being a part of the world. I go into a different dimension where I don't feel [physically and emotionally], and I am not associated at all with what is happening. I disappear. For example, when I couldn't put both feet on the ground during an exercise it was because it gave me the sensation of being completely on earth's ground and I always wanted at least one foot off the ground, so I was partly in "my place, my world." [When I do this] it's more than a distraction, it is literally [a way to] remove myself from the world.

As the group progressed, Rosalita's tolerance for being aware of what she was feeling physically and emotionally in the present moment increased through the consistent practice of interoception and choice-making. The ability to make her own autonomous decisions about what she wanted to do (what she wanted to pay attention to, how she wanted to move and breathe) during the yoga practice led to a heightened sense of agency and empowerment. Within the TCTSY practice, Rosalita honored her personal boundaries by choosing to either stop doing particular movements or diminish their intensity. Regarding her process for making decisions during the yoga practice, Rosalita said,

It's almost like you know your limitations. Sometimes it would become really overwhelming and I wasn't about to stay there . . . It's like, I know what's comfortable for me right now and this isn't it.

I was curious to learn more about how Rosalita understood and experienced discomfort. For example, taking her arms above her shoulders was a movement that Rosalita was often not interested in exploring during the yoga practice. For her, and for almost all group members, being able to make the choice not to do a particular movement during the yoga practice was empowering. Rosalita spoke about this at her initial interview.

For me . . . having the opportunity to say "No" was very useful . . . [In relation to] raising my arms, I always kept them at shoulder level or lower . . . I just couldn't raise my arms all the way up . . . I tried it

several times. It was completely uncomfortable—I don't know why. [The yoga practice] gave me a chance to see what felt right to me . . . and I had a choice. It's like, "Okay, if it makes me feel uncomfortable, I don't have to do it."

Recognizing the way physical sensations can inform our awareness of emotional states, I wondered whether Rosalita understood sensations associated with raising her arms as purely physical discomfort (for example, a pinching feeling in her shoulder) or emotional discomfort, or both physical and emotional in nature. When I inquired about this, Rosalita responded,

Emotional, definitely emotional. It was kind of like a sick to my stomach feeling. Like, "No, that does not feel good. It's making me anxious." Literally kind of sick to my stomach. There were a couple of times when I thought that I might pass out, so it was definitely emotional.

As the group progressed, I observed that Rosalita along with other group members developed an interest in exploring movements that had previously been intolerable. Some examples included forms that began in a prone or supine position, stretching arms above shoulder height, and holding particular forms for a longer amount of time. Participants also found that they were more able to make choices that aligned with their preferences, such as exerting less intensely, doing an alternate movement that was different from what I was demonstrating, and deciding to rest for a portion of the yoga practice. I asked Rosalita about her approach to making choices in relation to embodied experience that was difficult to tolerate. She replied,

Sometimes actually the [uncomfortable] feelings would increase, so I would go back to where I was. And then there were other times when I would realize, "Oh, this isn't so bad." And I would feel like I was letting go of those feelings, because I was pushing through. But I wasn't forcing myself, it was a gradual thing—because you never know until you try. And so that's why I kept attempting it, and I did! I had a feeling of, "Oh, that had everything to do with me."

Because there was never a priority placed on making one choice over another, Rosalita was free to determine for herself whether she wanted to move toward or away from any particular movement. In my instructions, I often made statements like, "There is no right and wrong regarding this choice" and "You are in charge of your own body; the choices you make are up to you." I wondered how Rosalita understood the value of being offered options that she rejected, and I inquired about this during her second interview.

RS: *I'm curious [about your perspective on this] . . . what if I had never offered that option to bring your arms over your head and everything felt okay to you? Do you think there was a value to having something offered as a possibility that just didn't feel right for you?*

Rosalita: *Yes. Because [saying] "No, that's not comfortable. I'm going to get to where I'm comfortable" [is] a way of speaking for yourself . . . [I learned that] I can say "No."*

Over time, Rosalita noticed that she was more able to remain attentive to what was happening in the moment instead of withdrawing during group sessions. Without any prompting to apply learning that took place during group sessions, Rosalita noticed that her growth organically carried over into situations she encountered in daily life. She felt increasingly empowered to voice her opinions, assert her boundaries, and influence her life circumstances. As a result, she experienced a deeper sense of connection with others. In our first interview, Rosalita described how she might have engaged in our conversation before joining the TCTSY group. She reflected on how developing awareness of present-moment embodied experience impacted her sense of self and her relationships.

Rosalita: *Prior to this group, I would have been like . . . look at that picture over there, I'm part of that picture . . . oh yeah, I would lose it . . . so it's pretty wild.*

RS: *The difference, you mean, between how you used to be and how you are now?*

Rosalita: *Yes. [Now I'm] more focused, like being in the moment! I'm here with you . . . we're speaking . . . [I can remind myself to] stay here . . . and talk, and just relate, and connect. . . . [Now] I don't dissociate as much. [Dissociating] was really my way of saying, "I'm invisible. I'm not here and you're not there, so I don't have to experience anything."*

Rosalita reflected on her process for making decisions about the way she cared for herself in relation to physical movement and breathing patterns. With increasing frequency, Rosalita's choices led to self-regulation. During her first interview, Rosalita described being able to shift from a state of tension to a more relaxed state by becoming aware of her embodied experience and intentionally adjusting the rhythm and depth of her breathing.

Yoga [helped me to get] in touch with myself and how my body reacts . . . I feel like now I have more control over myself . . . I always catch myself not breathing . . . when I'm aware of it, I do the breathing [I learned in class] and it's amazing, like, "Oh, wow, now I don't feel that tense feeling. I feel more relaxed."

When I focus on my breathing, it makes a huge difference. [The yoga practice] brings me back to earth. You know, I'm so out there . . . I can drive somewhere and not even know where I was, how I got there, or where I'm going . . . I am always so tense . . . [the group helped me] learn to relax. That's huge for me. And now I catch myself . . . like, "Rosalita, you know you are tense! You're not breathing! You need to relax."

For Rosalita, the yoga practice was an opportunity to cultivate compassion for herself. Building on a foundation of self-acceptance, she was able to experiment with following her own internal compass and making choices that were useful for her. During her second interview, Rosalita reflected on what she had learned in the support group. She characterized her experiences with the TCTSY practice:

In a strange way, [practicing yoga is] like accepting yourself: "That's how I feel and it's okay. It's okay if you're overwhelmed, it's okay if you feel good about it. It's all okay." So, you just feel . . . whole, more like a whole person, instead of pieces and parts. . . it's funny, no matter what kind of day I had, I left here feeling . . . more whole. Like there was some-thing missing and the yoga practice filled it up. It evolved each time to where I became more comfortable . . . and more secure, to the point where [I inwardly experienced] . . . "No! This is what I want to do. This is how I feel."

Starr

Starr joined the support group when she was fifty years old. She was seeking support to deal with the aftermath of a recent experience of sexual violence. Although she believed that connecting with other survivors of sexual violence would expand her current coping strategies, Starr also had concerns about becoming a member of the group because it was something she had never done before.

Characterizing herself as "driven, loving, and strong," Starr viewed the support group as a secure setting where she could move beyond isolation and discover new ways to address her trauma symptoms. Already in individual therapy, Starr thought that the yoga practice would add a physical dimension to her healing process. Starr reflected on her motivation for joining the group:

I wanted to meet others in a safe environment who had some of the same experiences I had . . . and to learn new ways, as a group, to help work through some of that. I was apprehensive about being in any group, but I thought that it would help me not feel so alone. [I thought it would add] the physical into my mental (laughs) . . . That's how I put it together. I thought it would give me more than affirmations or running my hands under cold water or changing the smell in the room. I thought it would add . . . more of a physical, full-body thing . . . that could help me . . . it would be a new tool to help me get through trauma. . . . We had all been through something, and we were all learning something different together. And that caused a [sense of] safety in itself, knowing that we were all moving through this together.

For Starr, one of the most important aspects of the TCTSY practice was the way her own internal experience and judgment were
prioritized. There were no externally defined standards to which
she was encouraged to conform. Starr became increasingly able to
use the yoga practice as a way to become more aware of her personal preferences in relation to how she moved her body.

Describing the evolution of her capacity to make choices based
on her internal experience, Starr said,

> [When I started the group] I felt alone, which made me feel unsafe. I felt
> like nobody was ever going to understand how I was feeling or what I
> was going through. Just being in a group of others that had been through
> similar things . . . the same, but different . . . that helped out. And
> to watch them being able to work through, with the yoga, the different
> poses . . . you could just tell what was better for them. I would be in one
> position and they would be in something totally different . . . but yet the
> same. So, that made me feel safe, knowing that there was no right or
> wrong way to do the yoga.
>
> I didn't know if I was doing things right, but then I realized there
> was no "right" and there was no "wrong." Because there was no right
> or wrong, I could do the same movements in ways that felt good for me.
> So, it helped . . . from the very first time, it helped. Once you spoke those
> words, "No right or no wrong," it helped to know that no matter how I
> did it, it was okay . . . That honestly was the beginning of starting to
> feel that I mattered again . . . what I need does matter. I matter. Even in
> this whole group of people, I matter . . . [the group] was the beginning
> of taking that back.

Starr reflected on the value of exercising choice during the
yoga practice and asserting her ability to accept or reject certain
options for movement. When instructing the yoga practice during
the support group, I often presented choice-making as a way to
say "Yes, no, or maybe" to movement options. For me, this was liberating because I was not trying to get anyone to do anything specific; rather, I was encouraging people to grow in self-awareness
and self-trust.

Curious to learn more about Starr's perspective on making choices during the yoga practice, I inquired about this, and she replied,

It was definitely helpful to set boundaries during the yoga practice because I had a choice. I had a choice to say "No" and have that be accepted, and to be heard. It didn't even have to be heard by anyone else, it just had to be heard by me. I was able to say "No" this time and then maybe the next time I was able to try it, if I wanted to. It was all very useful, because each week you feel a little different. You don't always come in with the same type of feeling. It was very useful to be offered an option. When it was "No" this week, it could have been "Yes" the next week. Maybe I worked through it a little bit and felt a little more comfortable with [the sense that] nobody's really watching me. Nobody's really judging me . . . nobody's forcing me.

Transcending rigid standards of "right" and "wrong" along with other group members who were also exploring options that felt useful to them during the yoga practice, Starr simultaneously experienced internal connection and connection with others. These bidirectional connections were accompanied by a growing sense of safety within the group. Starr reflected on the way yoga practice impacted the quality of group interaction that occurred afterward.

I definitely remember [when I started to understand what the yoga practice was about]. I think we had gone from the beginning, with everyone sitting around, to moving and getting onto the mats. And I think you said, "There's no wrong and no right," and something just changed. I felt connected to what I was doing. In our group, we were actually connecting in two ways. We were connecting with words and we were connecting with movement.

Until the time she joined the support group, most of the coping strategies Starr had used to address PTSD symptoms involved working with cognitive approaches to modifying her self-talk. Starr had also learned some mindfulness-based practices that emphasized attending to present moment sensory experience, such as olfactory or tactile stimuli. Starr discussed the impact of adding yoga to her repertoire of skills in self-care.

[A PTSD episode] usually starts with a trigger. So, I have a trigger, and that activates me. And then once I get activated, it's like, my focus is off, and I start to not want to feel what I'm feeling. I want to turn off what happened to me. I want to turn off the trauma of it and what I'm experiencing. It's always on this side of me [points to right side] and it's always flashbacks. Being activated is just trying to turn that [feeling] off . . . Being episodic is like, there's just no control over it anymore. I'm totally having a PTSD episode. That's the difference. Activation is trying to not feel it but allow it to be there. I'm trying to work with it from the present moment. An episode is just . . . it's hopeless! I'm there, it's happening. Flashbacks . . . like I'm there again.

[This support group] added a physical [aspect] to what I was already doing mentally to help me get through episodes. It added physical move-ments and a feeling of calmness. When you're mentally trying to stop what you're feeling, your stress level is rising, moving towards a PTSD episode . . . it gets exhausting. Adding physical [movement] to what's already going on mentally is calming. It kind of flattens [the stress] out and makes it easier to make changes on a mental level. Being in the group brought what I was going through mentally . . . down to a phys-ical [level], so it was more reachable to work on, instead of just totally going with the trigger and falling into an episode. It worked.

The yoga was more like a hands-on [approach] than a mental tool, because sometimes you just can't get there mentally. But you can do some-thing physically that will help your mental anxiety subside. It worked. It worked! I'm still using it. Sitting on the floor, with our legs crossed . . . we'd twist to one side and put one hand behind us to kind of push over . . . it does something for me. I can't really name what it does for me . . . when everything feels closed in and tight, that movement can usually break that cycle of that physical thing that goes on when you have PTSD. . . . The breathing's in there somewhere, too! (both laugh) I think the physical movement is what brings that strong feeling of . . . I'm way too tense inside . . . I'm way too bound up into this mental feeling . . . of what's going on inside my head. I'm way too bound up, so I think the actual physical twist opens that. But then, the breathing comes with it, which is kind of relaxing at the same time . . . so it just slows me down.

I was interested to hear Starr describe the way she approached making decisions on her own terms. For Starr, the process of choice-making was informed by her embodied experience. By paying attention to her body, Starr was able to assert her boundaries and move toward choices that were useful for her in the moment.

Child [a yoga form created by kneeling with feet together and knees apart, spine lowering toward ground, arms stretched forward with hands on the ground] was never something I felt comfortable with. I couldn't do it . . . it made me feel unsafe. Another definite "No" was downward dog [hands and feet on the ground, arms straight, and hips stretching up]. I just didn't do it. Immediately, when I saw what it was, it was a "No." I knew that inside, it didn't feel right to me. Thinking about doing it felt confining. So that was a "No." That's how I knew it was a "No," it just had that feeling to it . . . almost like . . . takes your breath away feeling. "Yes" was just "Yes." "Yep, I can do that! That feels good. I'm happy about that." There were no restrictions in breathing, or that tightness . . . there's none of that when it feels like a "Yes."

Starr also described the way she made decisions about sharing with the group during the period of time that preceded and followed the yoga practice. In a similar manner to how she approached the yoga practice, Starr learned to take her time, listen to her body, and make choices based on her embodied experience.

For a while, I just didn't even feel like talking. That felt like a "No" to me. I didn't want to say too much, I didn't want to open up too much. But I knew that, at some point, even though I felt that way, I knew that maybe that was in there . . . that I could get to the point where I could open up a little bit and share a little bit about myself, to feel a part of the group. At first, I didn't feel that I was a part of the group at all. I felt like, even though everybody else was there, it was just me. Even though I was interacting with everybody, I closed everybody else off. But I knew

that I wanted to open up, so it was a "Maybe." At first, it was, "No, no,"
I can't do that yet. The second week, I felt a little more comfortable with
it. The third week, I was able to just kind of be me, but when I was done
talking, it was like, "Done. Enough. Move on, please!" That was how I
kind of knew that "Maybe" feeling, it was like, "I want to participate, I
want to open my mouth and say how I'm doing or whatever, but I don't
want to let anybody in yet." But, soon, I just started to feel a little bit of
trust or more comfort with my surroundings and the other women, the
other people in the group.

Starr noticed that she frequently experienced a shift in the quality of her emotional states when she practiced yoga. Describing this
phenomenon, Starr noted that she also observed similar transitions
in other group participants' emotional experiences before and
after the yoga practice.

I remember [the changes] others went through before and after we did the
yoga. And I could actually see . . . and experience that myself. [My emo-
tions] may feel one way in a certain point in time . . . like they are too
much and it's too hard to get through. Then we would do some of the yoga
and . . . something like that can change my experience to become "Eh! Not
too bad . . . you know? This is not too bad." I did take that from the experi-
ence of being in a group and doing the yoga together . . . from beginning
to end, things can change. You don't always have to say "This is a really
bad experience, and this is how I'm going to leave," because it can
change . . . and it can change by a simple breathing pattern or movement.

[What was helpful to me was] remembering that there is no right or
wrong in relation to what I am feeling in the moment. I know that I keep
saying that . . . and also that I have choices. There are choices. I can feel
this way, or I can feel that way . . . or . . . there's a third choice! That
works for me. I'm not stuck with "This is what it is, this is what you've
got. You've got to deal with it." Instead of thinking "This frigging sucks,
and it's going to frigging suck," I can think "Oh, this frigging sucks,
but you know what? I can go over there and do that and I'm going to
feel better!" Because that's an option. Yeah, right now this is really bad,
you know . . . but something can change that.

Starr felt empowered knowing that she was able to take action to change what she was feeling, not only in the support group sessions but in her daily life as well.

[It helps me to know that I can influence] what goes on within me . . . knowing that I can make a change; I can make a shift. And any type of shift that makes me feel better at that point in time. If there are other people around, they're not really noticing that you did that, because people move all the time. It helps me to realize there's no right or wrong in where I'm at or what I'm doing, as long as I'm taking care of . . . what I'm feeling at that point in time.

Here is an example of how Starr applied her ability to take effective action. Going to the grocery store was often challenging for Starr. Sometimes she would become so triggered with PTSD symptoms that she would have to leave and go home.

An affirmation I was using in the grocery store before [experiencing the] yoga group was "You're in the grocery store . . . this is Friday, it's this time in the morning, everything is good. You're good. Nothing bad is going to happen. That's not him. You're good. Everything's okay. You're just here to get groceries. This will all be over in a little bit." That's the type of affirmation I would use in the grocery store. And I couldn't get there a lot of times, I'd have to leave . . . just leave my cart, and leave.

During the support group, Starr discovered that the yoga form called spinal twist (seated, turning spine to one side) was particularly effective in relieving physical, mental, and emotional tension. Starr continued to use this movement in daily life as a method for diminishing her level of activation. When she was anxious or triggered, even in the grocery store, Starr often chose to stretch in an inconspicuous manner.

Nobody really even notices that I'm doing that [stretching to relieve activation], but it helps me. It breaks that feeling of "Oh, that person's too close, they're looking at me" or whatever . . . and if I'm in the grocery store, I can stretch way out and grab that melon and roll it over (laughs) . . . I use it in that way . . . It still works, you know? Because it's what feels good to me. I can use it [inconspicuous movements or shifts in breathing patterns] in everyday life because there's no right or wrong in how we did it. "Let's stretch out this way, this melon's a little bit heavy!" Yes, I took it with me. For me personally, it moved mountains in my healing process.

Now this [stretching out and twisting her spine to reach for an item at the store] is one of my favorites [ways to address activation], so that's why I use it. You [might] see me standing in the grocery store like this (laughs), because the grocery store is very hard for me . . . very hard for me. But I've learned to work through that. It's a weekly thing you have to do, you know, it's a life task . . . to grocery shop, but it's hard for me. So, I learned how to use stretching and the physical parts [of the yoga practice] . . . because a lot of times I can't get that same effect from an affirmation . . . that I can get from a physical movement.

When Starr was telling me about how she used movement to relieve anxiety, I was curious to learn about how she made use of the body-based TCTSY approach as well as top-down, cognitive approaches. I asked about this.

RS: *It sounds like the physical movement gave you a different kind of lever-age . . . it was getting you to a place where the affirmation couldn't get you. Is that right?*

Starr: *Yeah! It changes your breathing. And changing your breathing changes your mindset.*

She continued:

I was very disconnected when I started . . . very disconnected from my body, due to the trauma that I had been through. So, being in the group connected me. I learned how to reconnect with myself. What happened, happened. It was a bad thing. And it disconnected me. And I stayed that way for a very long time.

I never really could feel . . . anything I was doing . . . I wasn't feel-ing anything. I was numb. And it connected me back to myself again, to trusting some of the things I was doing, and the way I was doing

*them . . . to take notice of what was going on while I was doing them . . .
simple things like "When I open that garage door, nobody's going to hit
me when I get it open." I could actually feel that feeling again, whereas
in the past, I was just numb. After participating in the group] there was
still the fear there, but I was connected with what I was doing. [I was
able to tell myself] "It's okay to open this garage door. It's okay to feel this
door handle, to feel the lock turn and the handle come open. It's okay
to feel that." So, it got me back in touch with the feeling of motion . . .
maybe those are the words I'm looking for . . . yeah, the feeling of motion.
And bad things weren't going to happen, just because I felt what I was
doing, the motion that I was going through. So, it connected me . . .
because I was disconnected.*

*When we were in the group, I never felt disconnected, after I started
to feel connected again. I just felt like I was in touch . . . I was in touch
with myself. I think it was about five classes in. It was about halfway
through, that I actually just felt it. [I thought], "This is happening! I'm
doing this and it's helping me." It was almost like, when you think about
it, it could almost take your breath away because it just felt like a relief.
Somebody turned it off and now I was able to turn it back on . . . and
that felt good. It felt like I was able to take something back.*

Wondering if, after the group's conclusion, Starr was able to
sustain the sense of connection to her body, I asked if she could
comment on this topic. Starr replied,

*The know-how. The know-how of feeling, knowing how to get to that feel-
ing definitely stays there. Because there are still times when I can . . . I
can go off and feel numb again, but [I am still] able to get back to
that connected feeling. It will always take me back to the day I realized
(gasps) "I connected myself!" It'll take me back there. [Participating in
the group] brought knowledge and awareness about myself . . . of what
I was feeling and where I was feeling it . . . even why I was feeling it.
And that worked, even when we were just talking. [I came to have more]
knowledge of how I was feeling when somebody else was talking . . .
and knowledge of how I was feeling when I was talking and when I
was done. [I gained] . . . knowledge in general . . . of self. It's that*

way that the physical works into the mental. That's how it affected me. Those simple body movements give you knowledge of what you're actually going through, because you feel it this way, or you feel it that way . . . It tied it [mind and body] together . . . and it opened up a new chapter for me.

PRESENT MOMENT

Gracefully Broken

Reclaiming My Stolen Voice from Within

Nicole Brown Faulknor

AS I START TO UNFOLD my story, let me begin by sharing that I stand firm in celebration of my resilience (which includes all negative feelings also attached to my story) from a childhood of trauma, including intergenerational trauma as an African American woman with a history that is stored in the epigenetics of my present-day DNA.

Surviving multiple traumatic situations throughout my childhood created an embodied experience of being under attack with no safety or resolution. In essence, I had never felt that my body was my own. It was this entity that had been painfully smacked, punched, beaten, kicked, hated, and neglected in my childhood. I hadn't really thought of my body as belonging to me. I lived as if things were not real, almost like an illusion. In this illusion, I tried to always understand my surroundings and responses in others. This gave me a feeling of "taking control" of my environment, the world around me, to avoid feeling overwhelmed throughout my childhood and throughout my development.

What most don't know upon meeting me is that my exteroceptive vigilance and tracking of my external environment bears my gift to understand the subtleties when called to educate, teach, study, or understand something in my present environment. My harsh and unloving childhood environments, from infancy through childhood stages and onward, forced me to develop a sixth sense. I learned to take in the most discreet subtleties of a room in a nonverbal and unspoken way. Perhaps this is a way that I taught myself to interpret the incoming information, before a word is spoken. It's like I have two minds and they are working together at all times. One is non-verbal and proficient at taking in information at a high-speed level, split second. In another split second, the other mind sifts through information and creates responses and language.

A hypervigilance that once kept me safe to stay alive and survive my childhood now bears my gift. It's an adaptive survival mechanism for a childhood from infancy to adulthood that was chaotic, helpless, painful, and unsafe.

As I begin sitting and listening to every sensation on my body—a fluttering around my chest, the pain in my left shoulder, the tightness around my throat and difficulty in swallowing with use of my throat muscles, particularly around my voice box—I am brought to an emptiness, a void-like sensation in the pit of my stomach. The feeling as though I have been robbed. Robbed and held for ransom while tortured in the very hands that were to love, clothe, feed, and protect me.

One of the voids that I work through in my personal practice is the notion of abandonment, not only from my own body now but from my parents. I continually neglected myself the same way my parents neglected me. I wasn't in my own body. I was protecting myself from the outside, which feels the same as trauma (helpless, disengaged, disempowered, and dissociated). As a result of my childhood trauma, it seems that I could not even live in my body and, unbeknownst to me, I left my body and began protecting her terror from the outside world. I worked in overdrive to find reasons to protect her from the outside world, almost as if I didn't want her to experience any feelings at all because the ones she endured created too much suffering and pain while alone, perhaps a survival strategy. In hindsight, a survival strategy to make sure that she wouldn't suffer alone again, making everyone, including the world, a threat.

My late father, Frank (passed away spring 2019), was aloof, cowardly, sensitive, loving, and carefree from all responsibilities, with his choice being to run and hide as opposed to love and protect me. My mother, Aneita, struggled with rageful psychotic episodes and substance abuse to bear her pain. My parents reenacted their own stories unto their children. An untold story trying to resolve the pain and suffering of their own psyches. That made me an unwilling participant, resulting in my story: being one of ten siblings, born into poverty, raised in a small town, fatherless, isolated, and abused.

I began to understand my personal story from my own inner wounded-child perspective as an adult survivor of chronic childhood trauma. The severed parts of myself that were hurt, terrified, vulnerable, neglected, and never allowed to be expressed are my inner wounded child. Every time something inescapable happened in my childhood, I'd split off energetically and disconnect from the rest of myself to survive the pain. This severed part of me, which is frozen in sheer panic and terror and is incomplete, is my inner wounded child. My inner wounded child still feels like she is protecting me from imminent danger all the time, yet she now terrorizes me with her presence, signaling that we are not safe yet. My childhood survival system kept me safe, but it also imprisons me today, safeguarding me from the world and others. This trapped survival system, a silent terrorized past, lives out invisibly in my present.

I have quietly begun to learn to move through the traumatized parts of myself through Trauma Center Trauma-Sensitive Yoga (TCTSY), first by learning that I had a body and this body had feelings, and then by feeling my body and claiming my body. My body belonged to me. I began by tracking movement inward, as opposed to room gazing and trying to get it right, listening to the facilitator's instruction. I learned to stay with any shape I had invited to my body and to notice what happened when my body moved. *Did I feel fluttering in my stomach? Am I angry with the tone of the facilitator's voice? Are my thoughts telling me something by observing my thought patterns?* I continued investigating my body and the sensations, as authentically as I could. I was unhurried. I moved when I wanted to and explored alternative shapes with my body outside of the instructions. Over a length of time I began to notice feelings of what felt like embarrassment, competing with others, then trying to be invisible in the room as a theme. This led me into learning more about my body because I became curious about exploring it in each practice, asking myself questions like *What do I need right now? What is this teaching me?* and *What can I let go of?* I learned to stay close to my breath with each movement. I taught myself that I could be present without thoughts ruminating, if I kept close company to my breath.

Over time it allowed me to learn calming my body, feeling inside my body with the rhythm of my breathing, and giving myself permission to stay with my breath and my body simultaneously. This permission allowed me to explore parts of my body story that hold the shame, the secrets, and the unspoken. They came in the form of fleeting memories and bodily sensations that I witnessed while moving my body. There were stories that I had never shared, like the chaotic and war-like home environment, created by an attachment figure who abused her power (with the inability to empathize), which had my body bear the suffering of every form of abuse, including financial abuse and witnessing horrific domestic incidents.

Unbeknownst to me, I created a whole slew of survival resources that may have constructed a social Self, one that would remain in the limelight and would be made known to those around me. This use of my social Self became very comfortable for me, perhaps so comfortable that I forgot what it felt like to have suffered throughout my childhood. I may have been constructed in this particular way in order to carry on with normal daily life within such terror. Therefore, I continued surviving my life and did not know how to live it. This quiet and isolated side (hidden trauma parts), the side that I have learned to know through TCTSY, may have not gotten any "light" whatsoever and may have been severed from my social Self in order to protect myself from fear, feelings of confinement, and punishment. It was through the opportunity to explore sensations and notice what I might be feeling, in varying shapes and forms with my body, that memories began coming together to be witnessed, without the need to explain, prove, and defend.

Speaking of defending and protecting, I found that the biggest resistance to doing TCTSY both as a survivor and as a facilitator was my thought sensations. By *thought sensations* I mean noticing my thoughts—for example, intrusive thoughts, negative thoughts, paranoid thoughts—then feeling those emotions in my body. They would have me feeling so physically helpless in a class. I had to get through the thoughts first; then I began to notice that thoughts were sensations to notice and to feel too. Thoughts of shame that I felt in my body resulted in me not wanting to move my body in certain ways. This may have been a response in efforts to avoid this particular feeling of shame. The feeling in my body, feeling small and disgusting, made me feel like I was being judged; and the feeling of disgust, which made me not want to lift my arm as high as I'd wanted, this crippling embodied shame was a block—I eventually realized that others in the room weren't watching me, because they were having their own embodied awareness. This supported me working through this observation of shame. It was comforting.

Over time I began to extend my arm more and more and noticed that my shoulders hunched over in front of my body shamefully. Discovering at that moment that I had power and choice—I had full control and could choose to lift myself up, by lifting my shoulders and bringing them back and down—was liberating because I could take action to change the way my body felt. I discovered that I could experience the tiniest of sensations from feeling and noticing my shoulder movements. I found I could experience the sensations moving from my shoulder into my heart center. I had never followed a sensation around my shoulder blade before, investigating where it goes. I began tracking these sensations on the front side of my body. I could even feel fragility of my heart. It felt like a ticklish sensation around the left side of my body. I found myself coughing. I felt as though I couldn't catch all of my breath. Maybe it was my terror speaking or maybe the fear that's been trapped in my body—localized there. In the subtleties of these present-moment movements, I began learning to listen and to feel for one of the first times in my life.

With a little over two years of practicing and training in TCTSY under my belt, I began to facilitate TCTSY. I began to become familiar with more sensations in my body, and my body and I started to become friendly. I began noticing sensations and stories coming together. I noticed the hunch I felt on my body from the inside, which I termed the *punishment hunch* because of the curling under of my pelvic floor and rounding sensation in my shoulder when I am in my most natural state. The punishment hunch most likely stored painful childhood beatings with agonizing memories of not being comforted afterward; from the endless lashes with the belt; the cowering and helplessness from physical, psychological abuse and emotional duress; or maybe it goes back even further to ancestral embodiment of the suffering and pain, migrating with whips and torture during slavery?

I've experienced intergenerational trauma as an African American woman with a history that is stored in the epigenetics. With that said, what's the core issue for African American culture to begin to build awareness of? It might be the emotional conditioning of American slavery in the genetic history and a trauma that started with confinement and punishment, as well as a migration history that may give rise to pain and suffering. The frightful experience of being kidnapped, tortured, and sold against the individual will of a person runs deeply through our history, and I realize that my very own culture may still be suffering from the long-term effects of this resistance to inescapable, traumatizing enslavement treatment—with no opportunity to discharge from survival response. The trauma is not over. It is ongoing. How can we heal from trauma when it is ongoing?

During class one day, I noticed sensations around my throat, which led me to a story from when I was eleven years old and had choked on a jawbreaker while alone in my room reading a book. When I discovered that I was unable to dislodge it from my throat, I ran downstairs in sheer panic to my mother, who was sitting at the kitchen table doing school work. She noticed my hands around my neck and quickly approached me, bending me over and belting blows with her fist to my back in desperation and panic to help me. I was able to push my fingers down my throat between the blows and threw up the jawbreaker, which my younger sister quickly snatched up as "candy," popping it into her mouth. This near-death experience with no empathy afterward of a cuddle, a check-in with how I was feeling, had me repress this terror and memory until one evening after a TCTSY class this past year.

The evenings that came after these classes often evoked other memories through night terrors of awakening and not being able to breathe. I had recurring dreams of feeling the pain of being helpless and unable to catch my breath enough to articulate the danger and harm I felt. I'd be trying to scream/breathe in a frozen and frantic state, trying to bellow out, but the high level of this excruciating pain only allowed a gasping sound to come out—no words despite how much I was trying in the dream, leaving me per-plexed, confused, and frustrated. Again, these could have been trauma body memories from my DNA history of hangings, lynch-ings, and enslaving chains around my throat during slavery.

These historical memories were solidified by my environment in the unexpected volatile outbursts and whoopings that my mother would give me, for making too much noise if she wanted peace and quiet, for not completing a household chore to her expecta-tions. And the ostracizing amongst siblings for the entire day, being scorned and made fun of; watching the beatings of my siblings to learn a lesson that was being taught as a threat; the strangulation of my sister into a near-death experience; and the many lashes and raised welts all over my body, sometimes four, sometimes fifteen, one time twenty-two. I would count them either in bed at bedtime or when left in the basement, where I spent most of my time as a child. We were always put away in the basement once home from school, Sunday school, and on the weekends. Children were to be seen and not heard. Yet we were not seen. No one knew the amount of time we actually spent in isolation, in an unfinished basement and with so much pain and fear. As children, we turned this suffering into "playtime" in the basement.

The weight and shame on my shoulder, bearing my parents' choice, was never mine to begin with, another empowering revelation to encounter from within. With this new-felt awareness and a weekend away at a silent retreat this past summer, I realized that I've never lived in my body before now, for over forty years. Now when I practice yoga, TCTSY, or any form of mindfulness meditation, I have learned to love the sensation of being in my body and choosing what I would like to do there—it brings me such peace, stillness, and a sense of calm. It has come to be a "newfound place." My body.

The present-moment experience and appreciation that comes with being in my body: I can experiment and observe my feelings—I really love the movement and feeling of feeling me, inside of my body. I love stopping when I want to repeat a shape or form in my body. Experiencing a thought I might have been holding on to for a day or week and breathing into it brings appreciation. Holding a shape to observe what I want to notice, for example, by directing awareness to investigate the movement of the sensation through my body, is all mine.

This brings me to a hatha yoga practice I did at a local gym, Christmas 2018—and being told by a front desk staffer how upset a colleague instructor was that I was doing my own thing between her

facilitated poses. The staffer clarified, in a roundabout way, after
sharing my explanation for the movement between her facilitation,
that regardless of my need to find space during the Christmas season
and feeling down, it "did not matter because in this instructor's
particular class you have to do exactly what you are told during her
class." I felt robbed again—actually violated—that this instructor
wanted to do what she wanted with *my body*. This embodiment of her
perceived power and control felt no different from being assaulted.
To be invited to choose a feeling of helplessness by choice? I don't
think so. Not on this healing journey that I have been on through
TCTSY. The fear of punishment, known to my body, soon moved
to feelings of empowerment. Empowerment in having a choice and
that I get to choose to either continue to do what I want with my
body in her class or not return to her class.

I no longer had to feel the shame and anger of not being able to
do what I wanted, with the embodied fear of "getting into trouble."
They say when you are your own fog, it's hard to see through someone else's—my vision was no longer foggy. The need for control
and power to possibly mask a sense of low self-worth was evident in
my colleague. It had nothing to do with me.

The art of being seen has a powerful unfolding: the opportunity to
have my story told to me from me, by listening with my body.

My thoughts are a sensation that I began to explore from
within—the primitive survival response of intellectualizing as
opposed to feeling what I am feeling. It had been easier up to this
point to make sense of the world, from a very young age, when I felt
hurt, scared, sad, and alone. I could process my feelings by understanding and intellectualizing situations around me, but I think
that this became a response to not having to feel those feelings or
maybe try to make sense of them by myself. Why does my mother
hate me so much? Why am I such a bad kid? What can I do to make
her love me? No one ever explained anything to me as a child, and

I had always felt alone, unsafe, and distrusting. The frustration of being told what to do—the noticing that I cannot think for myself. The feelings of resentment were shared to me from my body when given the freedom to choose shapes and forms with my body, to be present, and to take effective action in the invitations. The learning to exist inside of my fragmented wholeness.

This learning to exist inside of my fragmented wholeness was me attempting to integrate this terrifying and alien part of my Self (my childhood trauma), which came with the realization that the wounded part of me had been unreachable—and had been armored and split off. With this new discovery I saw how I had completely separated from my feelings, particularly the feelings that reminded me of hurt, sadness, and fear, which could be most things in my adult world today. This entrapment came in varying ages with many different ego states depending on the situation at hand. Each part of my fragments seemed to bear different emotions that held their own complexity and stories.

I am on a continuous uncovering of my inner wounded child. It seems as if she has been woven into a weblike invisible structure that has kept her encased, and now we (she and I) must relearn everything. We are starting to resolve and teach our bodily networks, which appear to have been controlled by our traumatized brain, that we are now safe. We internalized ourselves to survive, and now we no longer know how to live externally because we are unable to think and act from this primal brain response guided by our implicit and explicit memories. I think that I have internalized the tormented parts of myself as a way to ensure that I am forever protected, which would be a guarantee to never return to the helplessness and despair that my body experienced in my childhood. At any given time, any given moment, I can be reminded of the mean cashier at checkout, the voiceless child on the subway station gazing up at their parents, the silenced man who lives homelessly on the street and has lost hope in society. All of these feelings, when I observe them in my "normal" day-to-day living, are reminders to me of my own story.

I needed to learn how to feel safe with others; I needed to grieve the childhood I received and the childhood I did not receive; I needed to work through my fears, shame, and anger as I realized that these emotions were never expressed—talked about but never felt and expressed—and may have been needed in order to grieve. It was left unfinished. Unfinished childhood. Unfinished love.

There has been nothing more liberating than *both* knowing and feeling that I deserved more. Noticing I had deserved more and I could give myself all that I had not been given. Noticing I was now giving myself what I needed and what I had deserved, from that moment of realization onward. This meant giving myself time; remaining unhurried; doing one thing at a time; being in control of my body; and responding to the body authentically and accordingly. This noticing has now turned inward.

From Human Doing to Human Being

Reconnecting to Native American Spiritual Embodiment through the Practice of Presence

Kate O'Hara

I MET EFFIE IN A treatment program where I facilitated yoga classes. Immediately I saw her kind and quiet demeanor and noticed how her huge, bright smile lit up the room. She was 100 percent curious, always asking more nuanced questions as if she were searching for something: "How can you relax when you can't feel your body? How do you know when you're in the present moment? What's it like to connect your mind and body?" I explained what I confidently could. I shared that through practice in class she might begin to notice internal sensations. When she noticed tension, maybe she could move toward choosing to release and relax her muscles. For as many questions as I answered, though, it seemed there were more that I couldn't. While I could tell Effie that feeling sensation in your body means you are bringing awareness fully into the present moment, I couldn't say when it would happen for her. I didn't have a satisfying description of what a mind-body connection feels like either. With a multitude of ways to detail the feeling, Effie would need to discover her own version. She was asking questions that only firsthand experience could answer.

Every day Effie rolled out her mat in the corner next to the door, choosing her location in the room. From a yoga studio perspective, this spot wouldn't be ideal. Her mat was facing in the same direction as mine but with two people in between us. During class it was awkward for her to see me so she could visually follow the movements, and I had difficulty seeing her. While I don't look at students directly during practice, I do use my peripheral vision to notice people's overall experience. Although awkward for me, I trusted that Effie knew this was her ideal location.

As weeks of class went by, Effie continued to lay her mat in the corner by the door. She was cheerful but not always chatty. Her smile was usually accompanied by a soft but confident hello. When she spoke, I noticed her eyes and their inquisitive spark. On a few occasions I'd wonder if she had a question. When I'd ask if she did, she'd give a quick chuckle and reply no, saying she was just happy to be in class.

When I contract with an agency for yoga classes, I often don't know the depth or breadth of a client's life or trauma experience. I might learn a nugget of information about their behavior, or sometimes a client will tell me a piece of their story. Details can be helpful, like knowing when someone is triggered by the sound of breathing, but often details aren't necessary. As a Trauma Center Trauma-Sensitive Yoga (TCTSY) facilitator, part of my role is to engage with people in the present moment, meeting them where they are on any particular day. If I know details about a client's history, then I run the risk of making assumptions about the experience they're having in a moment. I may misinterpret their willingness, body language, or level of engagement. I also run the risk of overlaying my story onto their present-moment experience. With Effie I knew nothing aside from what she showed me in class.

I had never done yoga before, but I was open to it. I thought it was more exercise and didn't realize there was more to it. It was something new, and I was curious. I wanted to find out more.

I put my mat next to the door near the exit with my back against the wall because it felt free. I needed to feel like I wasn't closed in or trapped. The only way I could find comfort was being next to the door and being able to walk out. I couldn't continue without it. It was the only way I could make it through. Having the freedom to walk out of the door gave me the freedom to stay put.

I didn't know what boundaries were at first. I didn't know at that point that you could be present or mindful. I didn't have a realm of emotion, so I could tell a really painful story without being connected to pain or sadness. I didn't know I had a body. I operated solely from my mind. I didn't even know what emotions or feelings were. I had no clue. I wasn't connected to life other than my mind. I thought humans just lived based on what they knew. That's why I strived to know everything. I asked so many questions, thinking it would get me closer to that presence of being. It didn't. I lived in my head so much that a counselor turned her head and said, "Do you know that you're a human being?"

I didn't know that as individuals we were called human beings. I was very intellectual, scientific. I referred to people as Homo sapiens. I didn't look at people as individual beings, that we had things that made us who we were. I had no concept of self. My concept of myself was what you told me I was.

I learned early on that Effie was the daughter of a Native American father and a mother of Irish descent. She didn't talk much about her mom, but she frequently expressed love for her dad and how closely she identified with Native American spirituality. Although Christianity has infused addiction treatment since the nineteenth century, Effie sought out avenues to redirect her recovery through traditional beliefs, occasionally sharing her present-day discoveries with me before class. She introduced me to *The Red Road to Wellbriety: In the Native American Way,* a book explaining how to work the twelve steps of Alcoholics Anonymous through a traditional healing circle.[1] When she felt forced to accept a Christian viewpoint in her treatment process, she voiced frustration as she set up for class. At one point Effie helped organize a powwow for Native American people in recovery, in hopes of offering space for the local community to be together. It was apparent that Effie was rediscovering her cultural traditions. What I didn't know was how deeply it affected her relationship to the present moment.

When my father was alive, I didn't know I was growing up in a bicultural family. My belief about myself mimicked how my father lived, and I didn't know any other way. Being Native American, my father was grounded in native beliefs, spirituality, tradition, and a way of being.

He taught me there's an energy out there, the great spirit, Wakan Tanka, that makes everything possible. There was no questioning it; it was just an automatic belief as a little girl. It's there and connected to nature, animals, and people. It was a calmness, gentleness, and endless love that encompassed my father. It's more about being in sync and flowing with that energy. Everything flows within Wakan Tanka. I had that coming into treatment. I was never tempted to not keep that faith.

When I was six years old, my dad died, and the synergy left. It was a way of being for me. I was old enough to know it and feel it. Without his presence, I learned it wasn't enough being me; I had to be something else. After a decade of addiction, I had to break through to get back to being in sync with the Great Spirit. Little did I know that this search for what I had forgotten would be found in a moment.

It was common that people came to class early for a few extra minutes of quiet, while some participants came early to help out. We had to move chairs and tables and sweep the floor to turn the lunch-community-group room into a yoga studio. On this particular day, Effie had been attending yoga class four days a week for two months. The room already set, I was alone when she bounded in. She laid her mat next to the door, her usual spot, looking like a kid in a candy store. She was excited to chat.

"Look at this! Is this a thing?!" She repeatedly and insistently pointed at an open magazine.

Effie was giddy as she showed me a full-page ad for probiotics. A cheerful woman was running along a park path, the picture of health. It looked like so many other supplement ads I'd seen, so I was a bit confused; was what a thing? A full-page ad? Probiotics? I turned my head with curiosity and a bit of confusion.

"Is this a thing all over? Do people do this outside of yoga?"

"Looks like an ad for probiotics." I was still confused.

"It says 'living in the present moment.' I've heard of the present moment in here, but is it a thing? For everyone? Do other people know about this?"

I answered, "It's a thing," finally understanding her focus. Effie stood on her mat, mouth open, in amazement. After a few seconds, she blinked slowly, trying to wrap her head around my answer, "I can't believe it."

I came to class early that day beyond excited!!! I was reading a magazine the night before. What caught me were yoga poses on the other side of an ad—perforated pose cards, one for morning, midday, and evening—about bringing yourself into the present moment. They were using words like balance, peace, serenity, health, and gratitude. I was drawn to them because I wasn't exposed to them before.

I had learned enough in yoga class to know the general concept of being in the present moment. I wasn't present in any other part of life but yoga class.

I remember asking, "Is this a thing? Do people do this outside of yoga? Is this a thing all over?" I definitely had no idea that the present moment and mindfulness existed. I still didn't have a concept that human beings had the potential of living in the present moment. I was looking at it as though it was a scientific concept, still living in my head.

I even asked Kate, "Does this come from the west coast?" The women on the west coast make good money, do yoga, eat well. They have their kale shakes in the morning, and they're living in the present moment. It was foreign. They were separate from me. I was trying to put a story to it to explain it. I was trying to find a reason to understand why I hadn't been exposed to the present moment. I didn't understand that my childhood played a part.

I was excited to be reading this in a magazine available to me. It was the feeling of God doing for me what I couldn't do for myself. Such relief. It meant that this was a part of the world greater than myself. I couldn't fathom that idea. In that moment, I still felt like I wasn't exposed to it because there was something wrong with me, but the ad made me feel so alive.

Reading this magazine, I thought, Kate is telling the truth. This is real. From this point on, I had complete trust in her. This was my turning point.

Yoga became my time to practice everything I had learned about being present. I could tolerate a minute of silence. Stillness helped define the peace. My body automatically on its own knew how to find quiet and stillness, but my consciousness wasn't connected to that. My mind never stopped. That minute of rest is where I could connect my mind and body. I was just being. In that moment, I practiced going from a human doing to a human being. That minute in yoga class, I felt for a split second like a human being.

Five months later Effie came to class as usual except she didn't say hello. Although curious, it was how she showed up that day, so I respected her space. We began practice in our usual way, seated warm-ups for the spine. First we moved through neck stretches, gradually arching and rounding our back. Then, we'd moved our spine side to side in ballet-like movements, a class favorite. Some participants would say they felt graceful. Lastly we moved into twists. From seated or tabletop, people could choose their expression of thread-the-needle. On this day we moved toward standing. Some people transitioned through a down dog, while others rolled their knees to one side to stand. Because we had changed our orientation to the mat, we refocused attention on the soles of our feet. For some, it was helpful to notice the texture of their mats. As we moved into warrior, lifting our fingertips toward the ceiling, Effie cried out, "I CAN'T FEEL MY LEGS!" Hearing the panic in her voice, I leaned forward to see if she was okay. She was looking directly at me, consumed with fear. Her eyes were searching, maybe for an answer but mostly for reassurance.

"It's okay if you can't feel your legs. Sometimes that happens."

"Am I going to be okay? What do I do?" There was still fear in Effie's voice.

"You're okay. You can choose to stay in the form, or you can make your way out of it."

"Kate, I can't feel my legs!" Effie was insistent.

"What if you put your hands on your legs?" I reached down to feel my legs.

As Effie reached down to feel her upper legs, I noticed her body release. Her shoulders lowered, and the tension in her face eased slightly. She took a full breath in, and as she exhaled, she glanced back at me with a half-smile, "Okay. I'm okay." We continued with movement.

At the end of class, I checked in with her. Although she had few words, Effie looked calmer. Her brow had lowered slightly, softening her eyes. Although subtle, her shoulders weren't so rigid. They had lowered too. Effie's arms now swung freely by her sides. With her ribs expanding and contracting instead of her upper torso, I could see her breathing was now full and consequently slower. Her expression and body language indicated she was ready to move to her next therapy group. These started ten minutes after yoga. Sessions could have twelve to eighteen people in them, verbally processing trauma and addiction-related stories, so it was critical that Effie not be activated leaving class. From a more peaceful place, she would be able to participate in her next session instead of being triggered by it.

Although Effie left that day with a gentle smile, for the next couple of months, she'd sit crying softly, not moving on her mat.

I was bawling in yoga class and couldn't stop because in that split second, I realized I wasn't okay. Everything came crashing down into reality. I could see it everywhere in my life; it was crumbling. That's why I would rush home. In a way, I wanted to continue the work on my own. I found peace knowing that it was ok to be honest about the ugly thoughts I had about myself. The present moment brought me to my reality. That minute of practice in yoga class became not enough. So every day after group, I would rush home before my son got home. I would lay my yoga mat in my bedroom, facing the door. It was the only way I felt safe. I'd sit there for an hour trying to find that feeling. I didn't have a name for it, but I had enough in my mind. I was trying to figure out how to reach the moment in class where I had a name; I was a person; I had qualities about myself that made me deserving.

I could never do it. It never worked. I couldn't leave my mind or be present. The first time I could access it on my own at home was about nine months into treatment. I could connect my mind and body on my own.

Up until this time, I had been teaching trauma-informed yoga classes. Working under supervision to complete the 300-hour certification program, I gradually incorporated the concepts of TCTSY. Two days after graduation, we officially added a TCTSY class to the treatment center's yoga program, meeting twice a week. Our new space, a small, windowless room in the center of the facility, was the perfect size for four or five participants, a counselor, and me. It was a significant shift from our ground-level, windowed room that held twenty. For the first class, Effie hesitantly set up her mat next to the door, more alert than usual. Her body was still but her eyes continuously surveyed the space. Compared to our previous room, the lighting was softer, the room more intimate. Effie expressed afterward that the new conditions were triggering, so we worked together to explore lighting options and how she could feel safer in the space.

Although Effie settled into the room more, she didn't smile much when greeting people, and her movement continued to be subtle, sometimes staying in the child form for most of class. This was a new way for her to participate. It caught my attention, but I knew Effie was excellent at reaching out to her counselors when she needed support. For my part, I'd check in every now and then with a casual, "How're you?" receiving an equally casual, "I'm okay." We'd both smile gently and continue about our ways.

With the new class, we introduced a psychoeducation component to our hour-long format. We talked about safety, how we could co-create it in our space, and why it's crucial to establish in TCTSY. I presented a brief overview of explicit and implicit memory to normalize people's experiences of body-based memories. If I asked what people were feeling in their bodies, they'd often answer with words like *anxiety, fear, gratitude,* or *happiness.* So we looked at how sensation words differ from emotion words. I expected Effie to be engaged in these cognitive conversations. She'd always been intellectually curious. This time was different, though. Effie didn't ask intellectual questions; she was asking questions about her sensations during class and what she could do with them. Her curiosity had shifted from cognitive to somatic. A few months later, Effie shared with me that she'd write down the sensations, thoughts, and memories that she noticed during yoga and take them to her EMDR (eye movement desensitization and reprocessing) therapist. Together Effie and her therapist would use her insights in yoga to begin their EMDR session. Effie had found a treatment routine that worked well for her: talk therapy, yoga, and EMDR.

As our new class found a rhythm, so did Effie. At times, I could sense by her subtle facial expression that something wasn't sitting well. With her eyes closed, she would furrow her brow and tilt her head. Then she'd begin to move her body how she needed, her movements so subtle they were nearly undetectable. She'd arch and round her back or rotate her torso slowly and with intent. Gradually she'd choose to be still. Her shoulders would release and lower. Her furrow would recede into the landscape of her brow. Her breathing became soft, steady, even. She looked rooted to the floor but could readily stand at the end of class. Every time she moved through this process, the furrow in her brow became less deep, and stillness settled more quickly.

I could see Effie was experiencing a shift. Her cheery smile returned but with less yearning and more peacefulness. With purpose and thoughtfulness in her words and actions, a quiet confidence grew. Although she stopped asking questions, others in class asked. She'd quietly listen then close her eyes. At those moments, her shoulders would lower and her chin would tuck slightly, her entire body releasing just a bit. She wasn't searching anymore as much as she was exploring, her innate curiosity becoming a guide rather than a commander of the mission.

Putting place, time, and feeling to sensation helped to begin the true healing part. Yoga class was where I could intellectually see where all my healing was needed. I had connected to present moment enough that when I was doing EMDR, I could take those little sensations and thoughts attached to them and finish them all the way through. Everything I took to EMDR and counseling came from yoga class. It's the mindset and mind-body-soul experience that taught me each part is connected.

I had to get comfortable with all that pain first to be present with any other emotion. Yoga helped me become comfortable with painful feelings and identify where in my body emotional pain was. First I felt pain as hunger, so I would eat to get rid of the pain. I felt fear deep in my back and legs, so I would intellectually run away in a book or TV shows. I was running away through exercising and using social media too. I felt sadness and grief in my chest like I was suffocating. I felt worthless. Only when I felt all the pain, got it out of my body, and cleared pieces of it away could I have room for other feelings and be with them. It wasn't good or bad; it just was.

For the first time, I felt myself using outside connection to feel better. I was needing to focus on being me, so I got rid of all outside self-soothing distractions, so I could be present with myself, to be mindful of who I was and my values. I took a parenting class. I cut off friendships with men. I dropped all social media. I put limits on Netflix. I stopped reading books and magazines, especially fiction. I stopped disappearing into characters in fantasy land, so I couldn't run. I had to reconstruct everything.

I put action to it sitting on my mat, just feeling and encompassing myself as a whole being fully connected to my spirit, seeing and knowing from my heart and not my mind. In yoga class, when the sensations would get really intense, I'd feel jittery, feel severe anxiety, pins-and-needles all over my body. I couldn't keep still; I needed to find immediate relief and wanted to leave the room. Intellectually I could understand why we were doing what we were doing, so I chose to stay on my mat. I needed to experience uncomfortable feelings, good, bad, or indifferent. It was my choice to sit when sensations were fighting back to leave.

I had two choices: life or death, to be a human being or a human doing.

The *Collins Dictionary* states that "being is existence," listing *reality*, *presence*, and *life* as synonyms. By this definition, our inherent connection to the present moment is clear.[2] To live as a human being is to live in present reality. Living in the present moment is existence.

How do we do this, though: live in presence? In TCTSY we practice being in the present moment by noticing our *internal* felt sensations, a skill known as interoception. Being able to feel sensation, to know we're stretching a muscle or we're hungry, gives us proof of reality right here, right now, and that we're part of it. It lets us know we exist and that we're real. To be useful as a TCTSY facilitator, I need to be present, sensing not only my own internal experience but also the experience of participants. While I can't know what anyone's internal felt sense is, I can attune to the energy in the room. I can notice each individual's breathing, body language, movement, and occasional comment. Responding appropriately to what I see creates an opportunity for people to safely connect with their internal sensations in their way and in their time.

Like Effie experienced, this process connects mind and body. It was part of her roadmap from human doing to human being: feel sensation, become present, reconnect to self. As Effie continued down this path, she would discover that being present could connect more than her mind and body but her soul too. She would discover that, for her, existence and a mind-body-soul connection go hand in hand.

Two years into our practice together, Effie found her aha moment. On what I thought would be a particularly nondescript day, she was the only client who came to class, joining our regular staff facilitator and me. The three of us knew each other well, so we chatted for a bit with effortless comfort. Effie seemed especially happy.

> I was in a place of serenity, waiting for class to begin. There was a sense of safety and trust and no judgment. Sitting on the mat I had this presence and connection with the women in there, with me, that I was okay to be me however I presented myself that day. It was a genuine love that flowed in the room. Practice started, and Kate asked if we needed anything specific for the day. I always looked forward to that. For some reason, that

little saying made me feel like I belonged. I belonged in this yoga class. I think that day we actually just winged it.

We started on the mat, slowly working out everything from the tip of our head to how we were sitting on the ground. We didn't stay there long, though. It was maybe five or six minutes on the floor. After we did downward dog, we came up, and we were standing still. Kate would always say, "Feel your feet on your mat and ground yourself and come to a position where you can look up." I don't know her specific words, but for me, it was a standing position of strength within myself. I led from my heart knowing who I was, where I was, what I was doing, what I was hearing.

Here she started sun breaths. Standing with my feet firm on the ground and sun breaths up, a feeling of being alive flowed through my body like energy. My body transformed, the energy within my body transformed, into a feeling of being a strong tree growing. Each time I would plant my feet down in between sun breaths, I could feel my roots begin to grow. For me, this was like building my values and my goals and who I thought of as myself, a woman of integrity and honesty, filled with compassion and love. Each time I took a sun breath up, my arms became the limbs to my tree. I was growing upward toward the sun. It became my life, and the way I viewed the world became endless, full of hope, and connected to the people around me in the room. It was beautiful. The practice continued like that with the warrior series, and I continued to grow stronger and stronger. I knew my tree was strong. There I realized that I can withstand where I am going, where I have been, and anything that could happen in my present moment at any given time.

Whenever we'd come down to the floor I knew we were coming to an end. I sat down, and we did slight, little movements to work out and get comfortable on the floor. Even though I was sitting in a crisscross form and my arms were right here, my spirit and the energy flowed through me as though I was still standing in this beautiful, strong-rooted tree. This is where the epiphany came. I could feel beautiful shooting stars flow all about the room. That's what I visualized, but that was the energy that it felt like in the room. I was just like, oh my gosh, I am here. I'm connected with this flow of energy that flows through all life. I could feel the love and compassion of the women around me with mine. It was a sense of peace and serenity. Everything became a full circle for me. It became whole. I realized in that moment that I was living and breathing in the present moment wholeheartedly. I remember my bottom. My bottom felt like I was firmly planted into the earth like I belong here. This is where I belong. I belong here along with everyone else because they all belong here too. I felt fluid and grounded.

That's when I realized I was a human being. I am real. I have emotions. I have hardships, and I have struggles. Not every day is a good day, but there's a lot of beautiful days too. There's people I can share it with who love me and trust me, and I can do the same for them. That's what encompassed being a human being for me. I am capable of anything. That was truly a great day. I knew I had found human connection. I had found me.

I am a human being.

Roller Coasters

Integrating Somatic Triggers

Rachael Getecha

One of the pillars that Trauma Center Trauma-Sensitive Yoga (TCTSY) is built upon is interoception, or present-moment experience. What is interoception, and why is it useful within the context of fostering recovery for complex trauma survivors? As neurophysiologist Clare J. Fowler wrote in 2002, interoception is "the physiological condition of the entire body and the ability of visceral afferent information to reach awareness and affect behaviour, either directly or indirectly. The system of interoception as a whole constitutes 'the material me' and relates to how we perceive feelings from our bodies."[1] *Visceral afferent* simply means that the information comes in from the external parts of our bodies such as skin and tissue and then moves in toward the central nervous system where it becomes what we are able to feel. Interoception is the "processing, representations, and perceptions of bodily signals," wrote German researchers Beate M. Herbert and Olga Pollatos.[2]

How do you know when you are thirsty? You first experience the feeling of thirst in your body, maybe in your mouth. Noticing the feeling of thirst in your body leads you to think *I'm thirsty*. After that thought, you might then choose to get something to drink to quench the feeling of thirst. Even as you are reading this you might be able to recall what the feeling of thirst in your body feels like. The first moment of feeling thirst—the moment of noticing the present feeling in your body, the moment that your body's sensation of thirst clues your mind into a need for water—is an example of the process of interoception. Coming to an understanding that your body informs your mind might be a different line of thought than you are used to. You, like many, might think that the brain is the sole entity that informs the body of what is happening, that there isn't a transverse experience of the body also informing the brain of what is happening. What we know through interoception is that we don't just have feelings in our mind that then inform our body about what is happening with us. We also know through interoception that our body provides sensations and clues that our brain picks up that then inform our brain to let us know what we are feeling. Imagine being thirsty without any sensation of thirst being present in your body. Would you know that you were thirsty without these bodily clues?

Knowing our internal states—the process of interoception—is an integrated and in fact complex operation. One key area in the brain, the insular cortex, helps with knowing our internal states. A primary job of the insular cortex is assigning emotional meaning to our physical experiences. What this means is that feelings and sensations don't happen in isolation. We don't just feel thirst in our body and leave it at that. We feel the sensation of thirst in our body, which then informs our brain that we need water. There is a link between the feeling of thirst and the thought of thirst. There is a connection between what we feel in our body and what we think in our mind. Oftentimes there is meaning behind the sensations; there is a connection between bodily sensations and the feelings attached to them.

What would happen if over time that connection between body sensation and being able to feel or make meaning of that sensation had adapted away from predictable and connected to unpredictable and inaccessible because of traumatic experiences? The brains of complex trauma survivors show either decreased activity in the insular cortex or an over-activation in this area. This suggests that survivors have dysregulation in the insular cortex, the part of the brain that has the ability to intercept or feel our present-moment experiences. Having little activity or too much activity in the insular cortex translates to either feeling too much sensation or not being able to feel much if any sensation at all. It also shows up in our bodies as not having access to assign meaning to the sensations or lack of sensations in the body—feeling it or not, but not having the words to explain or understand the sensation.

While working with survivors of trauma, you might invite them to bring awareness to a certain area of their'body—for instance, their hands—and a common response is either they begin to tell you all the things they've never noticed about their hands before, or they tell you they can see their hands but are unable to feel them. It is also common for survivors doing a movement to notice something elsewhere in their body; if they begin to experiment with noticing something like pressing their fingertips together, instead of feeling their fingertips pressing together they begin to notice the pressure in another part of their body. These are examples of how this adaptation in the insular cortex plays out in people's lives. There is a tendency to have a contrary experience taking place in the brain and body, where what you are feeling and what you are thinking, or the meaning that you are attaching to the feelings or sensations in your body, are not congruent to your current reality. This affects how those who have survived trauma experience the world—but also very much how they experience their bodies.

When you are a survivor of complex, interrelational, generational, or community trauma, you most likely have lived a great part of your life surviving out of necessity. When you grow up in a place, space, or community that is perpetually unsafe, you become hyper-aware of everything in your external world that could potentially cause you harm. For example, if you grow up with a caregiver who is abusive, you become very attuned to the times of day when their anger might be elevated. You become a master at memorizing their schedule and patterns so that you can find opportunities to keep yourself away from them. You become deeply skilled at reading facial expressions and body language. All these external or exteroceptive cues become the map to your survival. Survivors attune themselves to the external stimuli in their environments so that they can navigate their lives around any potential land mines that will set off the abuser and therefore cause harm. It is in this state of having to constantly be attuned to what is happening externally that survivors begin to develop the adaptation in the brain's insular region or interoceptive pathways. If a person is in a chronic state of needing to always pay attention to their external world to stay alive, the part of their brain that notices what is happening within themselves and takes stock of how they feel about it adapts and becomes more geared toward surviving their external circumstances. The space to make decisions based on what you are feeling internally is hedged out when your survival hinges on extreme alertness to what is happening in your external environment. In short, what you are feeling or experiencing in your body is irrelevant when your main focus is surviving.

While this is a brilliant adaptation that our bodies and brains make to keep us alive, it takes a toll on survivors later in their life. When you are no longer in the place where the traumas are occurring yet you are still completely impacted, not only in your brain but also intensely in your body, much of a "normal" life is sacrificed to the barrage of scattered traumatic residue left over from all the years of surviving. When we endure catastrophic and chronic instances of neglect, abuse, and negligence, those moments of traumatic impact ripple deeply into the far-reaching spaces of our minds and spirits, and then they begin to manifest in a multitude of ways in our bodies.

I know this manifestation all too well, as it was how trauma continued to unfairly impose itself upon me moment to moment and year after year, long after the traumas in my life had happened. I remember first learning about interoception and the adaptations that the brains of survivors make in the wake of trauma in the summer of 2016. I attended a training with Dave Emerson in Wilmington, North Carolina. I'm from the Pacific Northwest, specifically Idaho, and this was my first time on the East Coast. The twenty-hour training was spread out over a weekend, and after it was finished, the plan was to drive from Wilmington back to Raleigh, North Carolina, to catch our flight home the next day.

The weekend ended, and with Wilmington and the training in the rearview mirror, my husband drove us and our three kids back to Raleigh in a rented minivan. As we drove, I noticed how mentally and emotionally drained I felt after the weekend of training. There was a lot of really great information, and much of it resonated deeply inside of me. The research, theories, and the practice of TCTSY bumped up against my own complex trauma history. I felt gratitude for the information, but I was also highly aware of the adaptations that my own body had made because of the complex trauma I had endured in my life.

I sat in the passenger seat of the van, looking out into the dense, green North Carolina trees while thinking about all the newfound gratitude and awareness, as we got on the highway toward Raleigh. Lost in my own thoughts, I didn't notice the huge dark rain clouds that we were driving into at sixty-five miles per hour. Without the warning drizzle that we get in Idaho, an intense East Coast rain began to barrage our minivan. It was a complete downpour like nothing I had experienced before, it limited our visibility of the road, and it was so loud. The massive raindrops pounded against the van from all sides, and I began to panic.

A familiar feeling of anxiety and terror filled every part of my body, coupled with a strong urge to make it stop. Not only to make the rain stop but also to make the overtaking feeling of distress happening in my body stop. I started yelling at my husband to pull over under a bridge until the rain stopped, knowing that under the bridge the sound of the rain would lessen. The rain was so intense and the visibility so low that my husband didn't want to pull over because he couldn't see where the edge of the road was, and he was worried that if he pulled over the other cars wouldn't be able to see him there. He said, "I'm sorry, babe, but I can't pull over right now." He grabbed my hand and squeezed it tightly and then went back to driving. He had become accustomed to such moments of panic in me as a part of our lives, and in his own way of self-preservation he'd learned that his staying calm in these moments was his only slice of strategy.

That squeeze briefly pulled me out of the panic and into the present-moment contact of my husband's hand holding mine. It reminded me of what I had just learned about interoception. I remembered how during the training we talked about utilizing the understanding of interoception as a way to invite survivors out of emotional and physical manifestations caused by trauma and into the present moment of their experience. The training had time dedicated to walking us through various ways to engage this interoceptive part of our brain. One suggestion was to notice our feet on the floor. We did this by moving our feet back and forth and from side to side. Recalling this in the van, I thought maybe I should give it a try and see if it really works. So I closed my eyes and through ragged breaths and a racing heartbeat tried to notice my feet. I slipped my sandals off and felt the carpeted mat under my feet. I lifted my toes and then rocked back onto my heels. I moved my feet from one side to the other. I then began to notice myself sitting in the passenger-side chair. I began to move myself from side to side in the chair, becoming aware of the shifts happening in my body as I moved in this way. Then I placed my hands on my upper legs and began to press down. I could feel that contact and the pressure of my hands on my legs. I settled there and really focused on noticing that sensation in my body, hands pressing on legs. As the minutes went by, the external noise of those raindrops lessened, and the internal awareness of my present-moment reality became my focus. I was able to steady my breathing, open my eyes, and look up. The rain hadn't stopped outside, but the storm inside of me was quieted. My husband, who had become accustomed to the arc of my panic, noticed that this time it didn't go in its normal trajectory. He asked, "What just happened? What did you just do?"

What just happened—and what would continue to happen over the next few months and years—was the ability for me to choose to use this new tool of interoception. I had found a way of anchoring myself in the present moment of my reality instead of in the sensations in my body that were tied to the past. What happened to my body in the van because of the rain were sensations and subsequent feelings of panic and terror that were rooted not in the present but in the past.

The sudden shift from normal road noise to loud pounding rain signaled danger in my body—just as a shift from the normal noise of a late-night TV to a loud altercation between the adults in my family had signaled danger as a child. That quick shift in environment, although I was 2,500 miles and fifteen years away from the initial danger, took me right back to those moments in my body as a child when parents fighting caused chaos. The result was that I panicked and became fearful in that moment on the road to Raleigh, just as I did when I was a kid. I wrote earlier about how there is a tendency to have a dual experience in your body when you are a survivor: what you are feeling in your body and the meaning that you are attaching to that feeling are not congruent to what your current reality is. My experience in the van is how those words played out in my life. Time and time again. What I felt in my body—a shift from normal volume to loud, coupled with being in a space where I wasn't able to make it stop—caused the palpable panic. The meaning that I attached to feeling that shift in my body was that I was in danger and needed to find a way to make it stop or get out of the situation so I couldn't hear it anymore. All of this, the shift in sensation in my body and the assigned meaning of being in danger, was tied to my past experiences of trauma. Although my present experience was that I was in a rental van in the rain in North Carolina with my husband and my kids, safe and secure, my body and my mind were jolted back into my past.

This had been my experience for decades. Submerged in feelings of panic, fear, and terror, and ravaged by the memories of my trauma not only in my mind but also very much in my body, without any sign of reprieve. My story isn't atypical; this is what takes place in the brains and bodies of many survivors of trauma. My hyper-attunement to the shift in my environment was once a useful signal to alert me to danger happening in my home as a child, but on a highway in North Carolina it becomes an adaptation that is no longer beneficial.

After decades of similar moments, the difference this time was interoception. In that moment of panic, the reprieve came when I was able to utilize a new tool within me. This wasn't an external thing that I had to go get or an existential place that I had to reach to find solace. It was a new way to interact with my body in the midst of chaotic panic-stricken moments. Instead of my body completely taking over and carrying me through the roller-coaster ride of sensations and emotions, I was able to choose a different experience in my body in those activated moments. This was new. It was a stark contrast from what I had been wired to encounter because of the effects that enduring trauma had had on my body.

As we made our way back into Raleigh then onto the airplane the following morning to go home, I continued to reflect on my experience in the van and wanted to know more. I am someone who is always on a quest to know the deeper *why* behind everything, and this new aspect to healing trauma intrigued me. So I engaged in more training to learn more about trauma and how the bodies of survivors are affected by the experiences that we go through. I wanted to know exactly what was happening in my body in that van in North Carolina and why pressing my hands on my legs worked to pull me out of a panic.

Fast-forward a year and a half, and I'm in a more intensive train-ing program with some of the same folks who were in Wilming-ton, and I got the answer to my *What was happening in the van?* question. What I learned was that in that moment in the rain I was having a triggered response. Not in the diluted sense of "being triggered" that has reached pop culture as a blanket way to explain why someone is upset, but if we take a closer look at the common vernacular we will uncover what triggering means to survivors of complex trauma.

There are many different ways that a person can become triggered. What triggers someone is personal to them and their life experiences. The loud noise of the rain triggered a response of anxiety and panic in me. It wasn't actually the rain that triggered the activation, but the loud noise in conjunction with being in a space that I couldn't get out of tapped into a deeper traumatic memory within me. An internal and/or external stimulus can trigger a traumatic memory and therefore activate the response system inside someone. Some examples of external triggers are sounds, smells, body sensations, touch, people, music, words, lighting, loud noises, dates, and places. Internal triggers are felt experiences that happen inside your body, such as the feeling of abandonment or finding your body in a position similar to when something traumatic occurred.

When these external or internal stimuli occur, your nervous system flips into survival mode. The stimulus often transports the survivor right back into the moment of trauma—because it is reminiscent of the traumatic event—and their body responds accordingly. There are a few common ways that being triggered manifests in people. In the situation in North Carolina I was triggered by the external loud sound of the rain and the internal feeling of not being able to get out of the van, which manifested as panic or the state of hyperarousal. In that moment, being triggered felt to me like I was getting strapped into a roller coaster that I didn't ask for or want to get into. On this roller-coaster ride, I experienced an overwhelming range from feeling everything to feeling nothing. Being triggered is an experience of all-encompassing, intruding, and gut-wrenching sensations, feelings, and emotions swirling around in your body, and you have no way to get off the ride. Triggers come on without notice and often stay long after they are welcome. Many people can stay in triggered states for days, weeks, or months before they are able to come back to some jagged sense of normalcy in their body.

One of the most telling and interesting things that I've learned about triggers comes out of a study done by Bessel A. van der Kolk and Rita Fisler in 1995.[3] They did positron emission tomography (PET) scans on survivors of trauma to see what might happen in their brains when they reheard their own trauma story. The researchers had the survivors write out an account of a traumatic incident that happened to them. They organized the story as a narrative starting with a moment before the trauma happened, then the trauma itself, and then something that happened after the trauma. Their own account was read back to them during scanning. The PET scans revealed that the closer the person reading the story got to the traumatic incident, the more limited the activity was in certain areas of the survivor's brain. Specifically, there was less activity in the prefrontal cortex, which is responsible for behaviors such as processing, analyzing information, and making decisions. There was also little activity in the Broca's area of the brain, which is responsible for producing speech. The study found that in response to hearing their own trauma story years after it had happened, the survivor's brain, body, and nervous system responded as if the trauma was happening all over again in that moment. While survivors were recalling the traumatic experience, not only were their thoughts transported back into that moment of impact, but their brains and their bodies also responded as if trauma was occurring now, even though they were inside a PET scanner.

Reading this study gave me a glimpse into what was happening within these survivors' brains and bodies—and in my own. The implications of these findings are manifold. When activity decreases in the brain's prefrontal cortex, survivors are left to rely mainly on what is referred to as the reptilian brain. This part of the brain is primal and controls vital functions such as heart rate and body temperature—it is in charge of basic survival. Functioning from this part of the brain is often called survival mode. When you are in survival mode you aren't thinking or analyzing any information, but rather you are in the nervous system response of fight, flight, freeze, or fawn, and your main objective is to stay alive. The reality for survivors of trauma is that they find themselves in this nervous system response frequently if not always. If you are in a situation where you are chronically unsafe or abused, you have a constant and chronic activation of this response system. Over a lifetime, this sustained activation leaves deep and lasting adaptation in the brain, body, and nervous system. Kerry Ressler, chief scientific officer at McLean Hospital and professor of psychiatry at Harvard Medical School, speaks to this:

> There is evidence that chronic (persistent) stress may actually rewire your brain. Scientists have learned that animals that experience prolonged stress have less activity in the parts of their brain that handle higher-order tasks—for example, the prefrontal cortex—and more activity in the primitive parts of their brain that are focused on survival, such as the amygdala. It's much like what would happen if you exercised one part of your body and not another. The part that was activated more often would become stronger, and the part that got less attention would get weaker. This is what appears to happen in the brain when it is under continuous stress: it essentially builds up the part of the brain designed to handle threats, and the part of the brain tasked with more complex thought takes a back seat.[4]

Think about if you worked out only one arm for twenty years— what would the rest of your body not only look like, but feel like? You would have significant strength in that one arm, but the rest of your body might become weaker or possibly lose full functionality. This is essentially what happens in the brains of survivors, and it's what happened to me. When all you know is persistent danger, abuse, oppression, or chaos, you stay in that reptilian part of the brain, you stay in survival mode, and everything becomes a threat to you. When you live in a dangerous situation, being able to accurately and quickly perceive threats is a brilliant and helpful adaptation of the brain in response to trauma. But when I'm in a rainstorm in a van in North Carolina and I'm now unable to tap into my prefrontal cortex to say to myself *This is a rainstorm, your husband is driving, you are safe, and you're going to be okay*, that previously helpful adaptation becomes a hindrance when I get stuck in a state of triggered panic and fear.

I tapped into a traumatic memory that moved me into the fight, flight, freeze, or fawn nervous system response that internally is screaming *DANGER! You have to get out of here now or you will get hurt again!* When this happens inside someone's body, they have an inability to pause and accurately process what is happening. They move into a primal space of surviving where everything is heightened and everyone is a threat. Survivors can spend a lifetime in this space, moving in and out of varied states of being triggered, feeling like their lives and the lives of those around them are one second away from imminent danger and that no one can be trusted, continuously limiting their lives and social circles to try to mitigate all possible triggers. When your internal infrastructure is survival and that is all you know, it can feel seemingly impossible to escape this up-and-down cycle of existing. One can see how spending a lifetime primarily using the survival part of the brain and nervous system would create a strong inclination toward responding to people and situations from a place of survival. As a survivor you are aware that the way you respond and move through life is in contrast to those around you. You live daily with a deep knowing that there is something maddening about the roller coaster you are on, but you find "normal" to be unreachable.

Another compounding factor, but one that I found to be a key in unlocking my own experience as a survivor, also came from the PET scan study. The findings highlighted that the Broca's area in the brains of survivors showed decreased or little activity in response to hearing their own story. The Broca's area generates language. So during a triggered response or even during a traumatic event, someone can understand words but might struggle to put their own words together in speech. When someone is triggered, they oftentimes will find it difficult if not impossible to explain their internal states. So it's often unhelpful to ask someone to produce words to explain what they are feeling or what is happening during a triggered response, or ask them to tell you what happened during a trauma. You would be asking someone to access a part of their brain that isn't available at that moment. This plays out within the body of a survivor, where there is a deep well of knowing and feeling the atrocities that have occurred but an abstruse inability to find the words to explain it all. In that van I can see that I am having an intensely different response to the rainstorm than my husband and children are, but the only thing I can feel or think about is that I am in danger. I can't tell you why or how, but everything inside of me is screaming *Make this stop!* When the nervous system is triggered and you are on high alert, language to describe what is happening inside of you is oftentimes unattainable.

So what happens to someone who knows that something horrific has happened to them but is unable to talk about it? Or when someone has a host of disruptive behaviors yet is unable to moderate those behaviors or process them through talk therapy? What is left in terms of help or therapy when a survivor isn't able to process trauma, talk about trauma, and is in a chronic fight, flight, freeze, or fawn response? These questions have led many to explore interventions that move away from the top-down (talking) approach and instead work first with what the body is experiencing. In this bottom-up approach to interacting with trauma, there is an opportunity to provide choices to survivors that may change what they are experiencing in their bodies. They can move away from the dictated, ingrained, and overpowering effects of trauma and into something new, something that is their choice. This approach—acknowledging that the body has real and present impacts because of the trauma the person endured—is a shift from the traditional idea that if a person

talks about trauma, they will heal from trauma. Many survivors who
have reached out to traditional therapies are left feeling discouraged and unchanged. This is where I was at in the van in 2016. For
decades I had been suffering from crippling anxiety, chronic pain,
and constant triggers. I had tried everything from counseling to crys-
tals, I had been doing yoga for four years, yet none of it addressed
what was actively happening in my body. The trauma had stopped a
decade earlier, but my life was still supremely controlled by the rip-
pling effects that years of trauma had on my body. I was accustomed
to the roller-coaster ride masquerading as my life yet still hoped that
someday, in some way, I would be able to make it stop.

That weekend in Wilmington and the trainings thereafter began to
poke holes in my internal infrastructure, which was built on surviving, and began to shine a light onto my internal and external tribu-
lations. Instead of just being told to talk about or medicate away my
symptoms, I started to understand why my life had unfolded and
adapted in the contorted, anarchic way that it had. Science, theory,
and research explained and brought into focus my life experiences.
It wasn't just science, theory, and research for me but a confirma-
tion and validation to a lifetime of harrowing co-occurrences.

Most of all, it gave me a new tool, a pause button for that tired
yet familiar roller coaster I had been on thousands of times. That
moment in the van was the first time in my life that I had an option
to choose another experience for my body, to choose to interrupt
the roller coaster. In that space where I was able to pause and
notice where I was in the present moment, I was able to bring my
awareness away from the trauma, away from the trigger that teth-
ered me to my past, and move toward the reality of what was actually happening to me in that moment. When I was able to say to
myself *What does the carpet feel like on my feet?* and then from there
to really notice the pressure of my hands on my upper legs, that is
a moment I remember so well because it was a moment of choice

for me. Choice is something that seems so small, but when you are someone who has lived in a body that feels held hostage to your past, the power to choose is huge. Receiving that power to choose *not* to be held hostage in that moment shifted inherent dynamics within me. The option of being able to choose something different in my body at a time of triggered panic was a pivotal point for me. It was the difference between being strapped to a roller coaster that I didn't want to be on, with no control of when it started or stopped, and having access to the pause button and gaining the power to stop the roller coaster, unstrap myself, and get off as I'd like.

This practice of pausing and noticing my body in moments of being triggered continued to take time, patience, and practice on my part. That instance in the van was the first of numerous and ongoing moments like it. But I've learned not only to just take out my new tool as needed but to begin to implement pausing and noticing myself in the present moment regularly. This implementation of interoception and experiencing the present moment was so novel for me at first. I had spent all the years of my life in a maze of sorts, always limited and always fearful about what might be around the next corner. I was shrinking myself and my life in an attempt to mitigate all potential threats—thinking that if I just stayed small maybe the pain would stop or go away, but always living in what had happened to me. To have a new choice in my body was empowering. To be able to choose being in the present moment instead of being dragged back into my past was like breathing fresh mountain air after a lifetime in the smog. It wasn't that the triggers stopped all of a sudden or that in a snap all of my trauma was taken away, but amidst all of that I was able to find peace in the present moment and know in that moment that I was okay. It took consistent effort and practice to relearn how to encounter the triggers and stressors in my life. Every time that tether tugged at my ankle, attempting to pull me back into that unfriendly place, I was able to choose to pause, notice, and root myself into my present moment. As the years went on, that consistent effort became a habit, and I was eventually able to choose to stop getting on the roller coaster altogether.

Inside Out

My Felt Experience

Cynthia Cameron

DESCRIBING THE EXPERIENCE OF HOW complex trauma manifests in the body—my body—is difficult. I offer this as one experience and not a paradigm for all complex trauma survivors. My hope is that these words will open a door for compassion, understanding, and kindness.

I am sixty-one years old and was abused as a small child through my early teens. I was also the victim of a random stranger shooting in my young adulthood. Even now, after all these years, I wake up each morning with my hands in fists, my fingernails digging in to my palms, my toes curled so tight that they ache. I take each day as it comes and am glad for each day's chance to be here. So I release my fingers, one by one, feel them softening, notice and release my toes until I can wiggle them. Then I notice my heartbeat and breath. I take ten slow breaths to lift the tension and anxiety—some mornings it takes several tries before I can make it through to ten, be where I am, notice daylight in the window—and then I get out of bed.

As a child raised in a violent home, I was sexually abused in school, at home, in the home of family. I was the victim of violence in so many places that, even now, any human engagement carries the potential underside of abandonment or violence. My abusers were adults who were supposed to have my welfare in mind: my grandfather, a school

employee, a boyfriend of my mother's. This abuse was encased in
the very violent, alcohol-fueled relationship between my mother
and father. All these people were very kind to me at times—a piece
of toast smothered in homemade jam, a hot bubble bath, a new
tricycle, a bedtime story or nursery rhyme, a drive to pick berries in
the countryside, a proffered stick of gum, a compliment, "you look
pretty"—these all became predictors of, and appeasements for, violence. They were part of an intricate weave that inevitably was punc-
tuated by rape or other physical, emotional violence.

> I am at my grandmother's house—maybe six years old. It is
> summer, and I am standing on a stool in front of the stove,
> stirring a copper-bottomed pot of gently simmering Saska-
> toon berries sweetened with cups and cups of sugar. I can
> still feel the worn wooden handle of the spoon, smell the
> deep purple berries in sugar. My grandmother's voice is
> kind; her manner with me was always gentle. She shows me
> how to stir in one direction and to watch for a particular
> pattern that the bubbles make when the berries and sugar
> transform into jam. She lets me taste from a teaspoon. It's
> delicious. The berries were picked earlier in the morning. I
> have no memory of the picking, but I do of the ride to the
> countryside with my grandparents. I remember my grand-
> mother leaving the car, bucket in hand, in her shorts and
> scarf, framed by the morning sunlight shining through the
> trees. I don't recall leaving the car, but I can recall in partic-
> ular detail the soft, nubby texture of the tan-colored back
> seat cover, the curve of the inside roof of the car. When we
> got back from berry picking, my grandmother poured me a
> bubble bath, before we made jam. Then we made lunch—it
> was always cream of tomato soup. We ate our soup, and then
> my grandfather let me help him roll cigarettes. I remember
> the smell of the fresh tobacco and the feel of the cigarette
> paper. I used to like being able to use his X-Acto knife to cut
> the rolls into equal cigarette-sized lengths.

My father, a war veteran like his father, once told me that he was always waiting for the bullet that didn't miss. A survivor of a shooting myself, I think I may have been the only family member he could relate that experience to, who might understand. I did and do. For me, in any human engagement, I physically prepare for the bullet, the fist, or the threat that might express anger, the silence that is a declaration of abandonment, or the predatory smile that precedes certain kinds of physical violence.

All human connection, for me, begins with an inner recoil. My body tenses slightly, my stomach feels a bit queasy, and my external sensory perceptions become heightened. I am acutely aware of nuances in voice, body language, minute facial indicators—a slight downturn of the mouth, anxiety in the eyes, raising of a brow, tension or uncertainty in the voice—all for me hold the potential of coming anger or distress. I am on constant alert, even now, after more than forty years. Every hello, every exchange with a stranger, family, or friend—they all begin this way.

Because my abusers used kindness to prepare me for their violence, it took thousands of kindnesses from others for me to begin to understand the meaning and intention of authentic kindness, and even more for me to understand that I was worthy of receiving it. Understanding kindness was like learning a foreign language. I have fluency, but I will never be a native speaker. I understand violence, however, the way a nuclear physicist understands the structure of the atom. I know it in my bones.

I am not violent myself—the opposite, by intention and nature, but also by design. My abusers were utterly intolerant of any negative emotion from me. I learned as a very small child to always express a visibly pleasant, calm exterior, regardless of the level of fear or turmoil I felt inside. The consequences of showing my true emotion were immediate and swift, sometimes verbal, sometimes psychological, sometimes physical. Rage from my mother, who had to endure constant fear herself, veiled threats from my father, direct verbal and physical threats from my rapists who both, when I struggled, choked me into submission. This latter happened so often that I learned to hold my breath until I passed out, because I couldn't keep my arms and legs from fighting back otherwise.

Who am I? It is the first day of my yoga teacher training. Our teacher asks us to stand, feet together, toes touching, stacking bone upon joint, joint upon bone, in what he calls equal-standing pose. He tells us to ask ourselves Who are you? Why are you here? He then leaves us in standing for two hours. By the end I am openly sobbing. Even though I am standing and no one is touching me, I feel hands on my body that I don't want touching me, and in between the spaces of sensation, panic, nausea, and shortness of breath, I feel terror, like a gale-force wind, screaming through every vein, every muscle, and scraping the very the bones of my body. I am unable to make the choice to move, to leave the room, to go into any other form. I leave my body and come back, leave and come back, like a frightened bird watching from the corner of the ceiling and coming back to save her chicks. I can't articulate any sound other than moaning and sobbing. I don't know how long I have been doing this. Who am I? At that moment, I am the embodiment of abject despair. When the session is done, I apologize to the whole class and the teacher for being weak. Although I am a distance runner, I tell them I am out of shape and need to practice my yoga more.

My experience in the standing drill made me feel so exposed—like I was stripped naked. I was the only one crying—okay, sobbing—all of the others were stoic and "made it." Being vulnerable in a practice seeking to groom invulnerability left me feeling like an outsider, weak, and somehow broken—in need of fixing in the eyes of the other students. Like many survivors, I do not disclose my experience to many people, and never to strangers. Physical practices, when they are extreme, can have profound triggering effects for me. I completed my teacher training, but I had the local suicide hotline phone number pasted on a sticky note on my office computer screen the entire time. I phoned seven times during the six-month training. I was also very fortunate at that time to find a very good therapist, grounded in trauma, and between the two I made it through and beyond.

Who am I? I am a sixty-one-year-old woman, a successful business owner, a mother of a beautifully grounded adult son, proud companion of a beautiful Belgian Shepherd dog. I am musical, creative—a sometime singer, sculptor, and painter. I am athletic, a yoga teacher, runner, and a bit of a gym rat, and I am, people tell me, kind. I hope that this is true. I tell myself that although I am very challenged to receive love and kindness, I can give it. I know that the love I feel for my son, my dog, and my circle of friends is authentic—untempered, real, and pure. This is empowering for me. I love; therefore, I am. I am not a broken thing, in need of extensive repair. The violence that I have experienced is not me. I am human, imperfect, but I can love. I am worthy.

I am also an insomniac—I haven't slept seven nights in a row in my memory. I sleepwalk, and sometimes, even now, I "lose time," here and there, although not for as long as when I was young.

Why do yoga, or any physical activity, if the effects can be extreme? There is a fine line between the positive and the negative effects of body engagement for me. The responses can be overpowering, but, if I have enough self-care strategies in place, they allow me to break free from the numbing effect of constant anxiety, lack of sleep, and dissociation. When it's right—and it mostly is now—I am closer to my own self.

I was emotionally and physically used in the service of others' needs as a small child. I had to suppress my own needs—even breathing—to survive. It has been a long road to reclaiming and discovering who I am. Physical, embodied engagement has provided a critical pathway.

After being shot while out walking on the river valley trails (admittedly, this incident of stranger violence was a bit of piling on from the universe), I began to run as a means of reclaiming a space that meant a great deal to me. I was challenged at first, but I discovered that with a dog I could run the trails. These runs gave me mental equilibrium, a place to feel my body on my own terms. I had no words for it but knew in my bones that this running was necessary to my mental health.

The birth of my son and his subsequent care were intensely physical experiences. With my infant child in my arms, I could feel—I could be present. To my delight, I found I could feel and give untempered love. Over the years running, yoga, and other physical practices such as training in a gym, for me, have become experiences of empowerment and self-discovery. At times they can trigger anxiety, or challenging memories—good memories too— but, if I am attentive, I can feel my own self, and *who I am* in any given moment. This self-discovery has taught me that I am, among other things, playful, joyful, persistent, and strong.

One of the particularly distressing outcomes of the experience of prolonged trauma is that it buries itself deeply, outside of normal recall. The memories that usually form identity are not there. Traumatic experiences are wrapped around the parts of myself that make me authentically me, and buried deep within my primal brain and body, with aspects and understandings of my self. As "I" navigated the nuanced, and sometimes deadly weave of violence and kindness, I learned to dissociate with dexterity. I also learned to present the aspects of self that I thought were wanted—that would not trigger anger or other unexpected consequences. There is a studious me who was top of the class; an athletic me who could run a mile and do anything the gym teacher wanted; a musical me who had near-perfect tonal memory and pitch. A funny, impish me—a trickster and a prankster— who negotiated the playground, and the creative me who spent hours in her room sketching and drawing. These are all authentic aspects of who I am, but I struggle to feel all these aspects of myself at once, and, worse, for extended periods of time in my youth and young adulthood I had profound, frightening, experiences of lost time.

I recall becoming aware of myself in the middle of a high school French class. I was fifteen or sixteen. It was the middle of the term, and all our books were open to a page in a middle chapter. The feeling I can only describe as jarring—a kind of "coming to" inside my own skin, like abruptly waking from a dream that you don't remember. I had no recollection of ever having enrolled in, or being in, this class. I had no memory of my classmates, the book, or the content within. The teacher, whom I didn't recognize, was asking me a question in French. I heard her as if she were speaking through a distant funnel. My vision was impaired—I was seeing everything through a limited scope—my peripheral vision was nonexistent; my focus was blurred. I did not know the answer. I was absolutely terrified. I have no other recollection of that class, other than seeing the low grade on my high school transcript. I have very limited memories of my childhood, elementary, junior high, and high school, and they are not contiguous. Not only my concept of self but time, for me, was fragmented. I had no frame of reference for this experience, and I told no one—this was just the way my life was.

My memories are fragments, like pieces of colored glass from a bowl that's been shattered and scattered. Some of the pieces are lost; the rest are out of order but very real nonetheless. I am a puzzle of experiences and responses that I am still putting back together. I know I am musical because I have great tonal recall and pitch, and music moves me deeply in my core. I know I am authentically athletic because I remember fragments of physicality, joy felt while diving over a gymnastics horse, flying over a high jump, intermingled with the sound of keys jingling in the pocket of my abuser in the gym locker room. To enjoy these aspects of myself sometimes I have to walk through a shadowy memory buried in my bones.

> I am in a café, with a friend. We are talking and spending easy time together. The music in the background switches to an old classic from my childhood: Crosby, Stills, Nash, and Young's "Wooden Ships." I instantly feel a surge of lightness

and resonance at the sound, followed by tears. They just stream down my face, with no clear memory or strong feeling attached to them. "I love this song," I say to my friend, but I can't stop the tears. "This song always makes me cry," I explain. But I can't say why. I have no memory of why, other than the stairs up to, and the dark doorway to, my mother's room, a faint smell of male cologne, the sense of a shadow.

For me, getting to me can be like walking through flames.

Like many children who have experienced childhood trauma, I tried to tell but was silenced. To protect the school and the reputation of my family, the truth was actively suppressed. I was portrayed as mentally overimaginative, unreliable, lying, and promiscuous. What I learned from this was to never tell anyone the truth of my experience, ever. As a result, no one knows me, not really. I have close friends who share their experiences of sorrow and challenge, but I never share mine. I am afraid of being judged, abandoned, deemed too broken to function in life or the workplace, or that someone may feel that I might be violent myself—that the perpetrator's violence has somehow been implanted in me. This is a horrible feeling. My therapist once asked if she could share parts of my story with her graduate students. She told me she would never tell them everything, as it was too traumatic. I have never shared with her all of my experience, as I didn't want to burden her either. Just as I am challenged to cause distress, I am challenged and afraid to burden others with my story. So I'm alone with the understanding, the meaning making, and the going forward. It is the loneliest feeling. It's not that I can't share my experience itself as much as I feel that I can't share my own journey through it. I am strong, resilient, and I so value love and kindness: inherent, authentic qualities of my own being. I am proud of who I am, but I carry a feeling of fear of being discovered and misjudged.

I am in the yoga studio—the studio where I took my teacher training. It has warm wooden floors, softly curtained windows overlooking the streetscape. I am scheduled for a one-on-one session with a teacher I like, a young woman, probably half my age. She is a wonderful technical practitioner and teacher, and observant. My goal is to work on preps for inversions; my shoulders are tight because I also do weight training, some boxing, and my work entails being on a computer all day. I go in expecting pointers and some information about setting up properly, possibly practicing a few progressions, and some thoughts and ideas for shoulder opening. She enters and announces that she would prefer to give me a restorative session. I think to myself, I must look a wreck, and I feel a bit queasy, because I am not fond of the static forms in restorative practice and am not sure what this will entail in a one-on-one, but I say "okay," even though I really want to pick her brain and use her technical expertise to support me to do headstands. I like doing headstands. But what I like or want is not on the horizon for me today. We do a few simple head and shoulder rotations, cat cow, child's pose, a seated twist or two. Then she gathers blocks, bolsters, and blankets, setting them up to support my head, shoulders, and back. She places blankets under my arms and a bolster under my knees to create a bound angle form. I am feeling exposed and am losing my ability to move or respond of my own accord. It's as though a circuit has been pulled; there is a gap between the feeling of being manipulated physically and my own response. She then begins to wrap a yoga strap around my feet. The instant she begins to bind my feet, my heart begins to race—I do not mean beat rapidly. I mean race—so fast that there is no space between beats. Panic replaces blood in my veins. My peripheral vision shuts down, and I am looking at her through a keyhole, unable to speak or move. My face is reflecting calm, and I feel the corners of my mouth adjusting to show a slight smile. I am quite certain this is her goal—to help me feel relaxed. She finishes binding my feet and then wraps them in a blanket and places blankets on my chest and arms to weigh them down. By this time, I have left my body completely. I am witnessing the scene from a far corner of the ceiling across the room. I see my body, bound. I watch her leave the room, shutting the door, telling me she will be back in about fifteen minutes. I drift in and out of awareness over a period of time that is immeasurable for me. I have no recollection of her return, of leaving the studio. I have no clear linear sense of time or memory for some days afterward, and I don't sleep—if I do, there are signs of my sleepwalking in the morning. Fragments, shards of memory, and comments from friends and work colleagues tell me I fulfilled my obligations and appeared normal to everyone. As far as I know.

In this session I was expecting and had mentally prepared for a playful interaction, and instead I received its complete opposite—the intention of the teacher was kindness, but the result was extreme dissociation and flashbacks I took days to recover from.

I am drawn to physical pursuits, both because I am athletic—this is a part of my authentic self—and because physical activity can provide relief from anxiety and chronic insomnia. Physical activity is a powerful tool for health: preventing chronic conditions, supporting mental, cognitive, and physical health. Because of my chronic anxiety and lack of sleep, I am at risk for dementia, heart attack, and stroke. I worry about this, and as I age I am experiencing a similar sense of the physical vulnerability that put me at risk when I was a child. Feeling physically strong helps me cope with a feeling of vulnerability in all spaces and places.

But, as mentioned, physical activity can be a double-edged sword. I prefer intense activity such as boxing and high-intensity interval workouts, and I love the more physical, flow-style yoga practices as well. The setting (such as the presence of men in the gym), physical manipulations during a yoga practice, or certain forms can all trigger dissociation and anxiety. I have to constantly negotiate solutions to find ways to heal that have a lasting effect.

For example, restorative yoga can be difficult for me because it is often delivered with quite a lot of well-intentioned adjustments and touching—these kind of manipulations feel the same as those of my abusers, before they progressed to forced violence. As well, the shape and sensation of many yoga forms are very difficult for me to hold for more than a few seconds at a time—child's form is one of these. I am uneasy when I can't see what's around me, so holding this shape is scary. Plow posture can also bring extreme distress and panic, because my breathing is challenged—I have to work to not hold my breath and to keep myself from passing out. Because my memory is physical as well as cognitive, holding any shape for more than a few seconds can often (not always) bring a deep anxiety, panic, or worse. I am more comfortable in a strong flow practice, where I can continuously move through from form to form, feel a sense of strength, and feel my breath moving. A strong practice provides me a way of feeling my body but not feeling trapped in a bound or static form. I choose classes with short or no closing meditation or breathing sequences, as I can often become highly anxious or dissociative during those sessions and be unable to manage work or normal daily activities afterward. As an alternative, for years I practiced walking meditation—feeling my feet, breathing with my own footsteps. I still do this during my runs, when the normal stressors of life, work, and relationships layer and I feel my anxiety building. The added bonus of an extremely aware, loving canine by my side makes this a really enjoyable practice.

I can now sit in meditation at home when I choose to, but not always. If I need or want to, I will often use beads or an old rosary—something sensory to keep me present in my body. I can get to a place of stillness, but this place is a reminder for me of how I had to adapt during sexual abuse. I wonder if this is a common place—this mental quietness—but for me the pathway that I learned to get there was driven by terror. So I often simply pray just on the edge of the deep meditative stillness. "May you find peace, may the road rise to meet you, and the wind be at your back. May you find company to share in joy, to comfort you in sorrow. May you be loved, and may you give love." These are the mantras I use to keep me from tipping too far, when the stillness I find is too familiar, too close to a preparation for dying.

I have learned to recognize when a physical therapy is worth the triggering and digging through embodied trauma memory, and when it is simply an act of violence to myself I am engaging in to conform to a cultural perception of self-responsibility, healing, and self-care. For example, I am often encouraged to engage in massage to help alleviate insomnia, tightness in my shoulders and back, and anxiety. I have tried several times. Lying on a massage table, with my shirt off, face down, in a closed room with only one exit that is blocked, while someone lays their hands on me is not healing for me in any way. This will never change. I am okay with this. To ameliorate friends and family who mean well, I often tell them that I have had a massage and it was wonderful. I tell my very kind and well-meaning yoga teachers that it was wonderful too, even when it is not. I don't mean to lie. I accept their kindness, learn from their technical skills, and recognize that my response is mine. They are talented teachers, not responsible for my past experience. If I choose a non-trauma-informed class, then I feel my responses are mine to hold and deal with.

I have been able to afford (not consistently) talk therapy. This was powerful in that it helped me understand the impact of trauma as normal given my experience. I had an open-minded, creative practitioner who supported me to explore beyond talk therapy through a physical pathway. Initially she supported me to manage yoga teacher training (and other life stresses), and then following that, self-defense, boxing, and mixed martial arts training.

I am challenged with the physical sensations in yoga, and in other physical training environments, on many levels. For example, I am often unable to feel whether a physical adjustment is too strong. In self-defense training I was often unable to respond appropriately— for example, I struggled to tap out when my body was at its physical limit. I was fortunate to have a trainer with whom I could disclose that I was a survivor of physical trauma and who was willing to work with me and progress incrementally through the training. During our initial boxing drill, I collapsed after throwing my very first punch and connecting to the pad; it triggered a powerful flashback—my fist became my father's fist, the pad my mother's face. Everything went black, and my entire body went limp for a moment. "I'm okay," I said and got back up. Over time my trainer learned to see when I was really okay, and when I might not be. I was safe to leave the gym out the front or back door, take a walk, or just breathe to reset, and come back or go home if I chose. I always came back. I loved the workouts, and although at times I had to do some significant reassembling afterward, the authentic me loves physical engagement, and I really benefitted from the feeling of strength in all the ways that are positive for any human. As well, I gained the added confidence that I could, if necessary, defend myself.

> I have my boxing gloves on, and my trainer is holding the pads. I am supposed to jab twice and cross. When I connect to the pad, he says in his gravelly voice, "SHHH, exhale when you connect, Cameron!" I can't make the sound. The skin on the back of my neck rises; I struggle to stay present. I do it again: jab, jab, cross. He injects "shhh," "shh," "SHHH" with each punch. I can't do it, my teeth clench at every exhale, and I am really afraid to tell him why. I don't want every single action I take to be defined by my abusers. I just want to learn how to throw a fucking punch. But I can't breathe the way he wants me to. I suck it up and decide to risk it. Before putting on my gloves at our next session, I say to him, "So, if you are a pedophile, what would you say to a child that you are about to abuse?" He looks at me. I can see the light

go on, and he nods. I put on my gloves and my helmet, and we start our boxing drills. I exhale strongly with a "whoosh" sound, each punch, and he smiles. "Okay, Cameron. Move your feet. Yes, Yessss!" he says when I connect.

I am very challenged to articulate discomfort, unhappiness, unease, or anger to others, even after these many years. I experience dissociation, sensory dysregulation, anxiety, freezing in many yoga, personal training, and other physical activity sessions. Still, for me, physical practices are very valuable, despite their challenges. Maybe it's meeting the challenge where it lives—in my body, more than in my mind—that works.

It is late afternoon and the sun is streaming through the windows that line the yoga studio. Even though it is cold outside, I feel the warmth on my skin. A familiar teacher comes in to the room and smiles when she sees me. She walks over and gives me a hug, which I reciprocate. I have known her in this setting for more than ten years and have watched her transform from young adult to mature woman. Witnessing, being a small part of her journey, has meaning for me. We begin practice as we frequently do, standing on our mats preparing for sun salutations. I am aware of the people on the mats around me but begin to bring my awareness into my own body. I feel my feet on my mat. The familiar ache of my bunioned, distance-runner feet makes me smile—I feel the corners of my mouth lift. I am familiar with the forms that we are engaging with, I breathe in, feel my ribs expand, and a hitch in my left shoulder as I raise my arms, which I roll out in response. I press my palms, exhale, wiggle my toes to stretch and find the base of my big and little toe. Folding forward I feel my fingers, still a bit cool from a chilly walk to the studio, against the rough surface of my well-worn mat. I stretch out to a half-lift, feel a bit of stiffness in my spine and the back of my hamstrings. I bring pressure from my heels and the base of my toes, engage my legs as I fold forward again. I breathe my own rhythm, checking in with my own body through the familiar sun salutations. I feel my strong, stiff, runner's legs from the back of my calves through my quads. I rejoice in my singer's lungs expanding and contracting, freely—I always choose to ignore constricted ujjayi breathing. I am a subversive, quiet, joyful, free breather. I love the experience of breathing on my own terms. This is my movement, my body, my breath, my rhythm, my practice.

The Disconnected Self
in Eating Disorders

Simona Anselmetti

I WOULD LIKE TO SHARE my path from discovering yoga for my own healing to my work as a Trauma Center Trauma-Sensitive Yoga (TCTSY) facilitator of clients with eating disorders. I have lived in and around Milan, one of the more modern cities of Italy, for all of my life. In my country yoga has become popular only in the last fifteen to twenty years. Twenty years ago, very few yoga studios were open, and the practice was considered something for "strange people," perhaps reflective of the cultural assumptions and judgments at the time. The landscape of yoga in Italy has changed considerably since then. In Milan at the moment there are dozens of yoga studios, and thousands of people are practicing.

I am both a psychotherapist and a researcher, and my path to become a practitioner of trauma-sensitive yoga started from an intuition about fifteen years ago. I had been personally experiencing how yoga improved my relationship to my body and the impact it had on my life. Over the course of time, TCTSY became embedded in my practice as a therapist and the central part of my research work.

Among the five pillars of TCTSY—invitational language, present-moment experiences, choice-making, shared authentic experience, and non-coercion—the one that resonates with my work in eating disorders is present-moment experience, which we explore through interoception, the ability to notice sensation within our own body.

It seems easily comprehensible that in a psychopathology where the disconnection from the body is the central aspect, a body-first approach like yoga could be very effective. But it is only recently that yoga has even been considered as an adjunctive treatment for eating disorders.

A tailored protocol of TCTSY for people with eating disorders doesn't currently exist, but sensing that the impact could be profound, I used the TCTSY pillars as guideposts, while also relying on my years of experience working with and supporting clients with eating disorders. As both a therapist and a TCTSY facilitator, I also incorporated detailed feedback from my colleagues and clients to help me thoughtfully integrate yoga into my work with eating disorders.

$$\text{\%} \quad \text{\%} \quad \text{\%}$$

I have personally struggled a lot since my teenage years with body dissatisfaction. I didn't like my body at all. Although my weight was perfectly normal, I never liked my appearance, considered my thighs too big, or found other "flaws" to focus on. Moreover, I wasn't very athletic or good at sports, so I also didn't have the chance to experience my body as functioning well; it felt useless to me. When I first found yoga, at thirty years old, I finally felt connected to my body. It was therapeutic for me, helping me be more calm, present, and finally centered within my own skin. I started my yoga practice in 2008 with a very soft hatha yoga practice in a small group of four people. After carrying the burden of feeling critical of my body and appearance, those first moments in yoga when I didn't feel critical about the appearance of my body were life-changing. For the first time in my life, I was only aware of how my body functioned. I started to realize that I was breathing and that I could control my breath. I started to feel my muscles, discovering that my arms were very strong and not only "big" as I had always seen them. It was like I was waking up to my body.

I continued to explore this experience until I got pregnant, two years later. I practiced prenatal yoga for the following months, and it helped me a lot to connect not only to my body and my breath but also to my baby. I experienced a deep connection with her. I was able to start listening to her when she was in my belly, and I believe that helped me better synchronize with her needs once she was born. Practicing yoga during this time was also useful for accepting the changes in shape and function of my body during pregnancy, which was very different from any other moment of my life when the changes of weight gain, different eating preferences, gastrointestinal distress, or back pain would throw me into deep self-criticism.

I stopped practicing yoga for two years after my daughter was born, until a Bikram yoga studio opened close to my apartment. That was my real falling in love with yoga, even if now I understand that it had several limits. At that moment in my life, there was a real change in my perspective: in ninety minutes of seeing my body squeezing and moving during the practice, not once did a negative thought arise. This process helped me a lot in accepting my body. After three years taking three or four classes weekly, two things happened at the same time: I learned about the sexual harassment lawsuits filed against the founder, Bikram Choudhury, and other violence he was perpetrating on people working with him (racist outbursts, aggressive behavior, and so on); and I started to find the practice of Bikram yoga too directive and not healthy for me anymore. With my knowledge today, I can understand that what we did in those classes was the opposite of a trauma-informed practice. Starting from the beginning, you were expected to expose your body in bikini or something similar because of the severely hot room, at least 104°F. Not only are you exposed in front of others but also scrutinized by your own gaze reflected in the mirrors covering two sides of the room. The instructors claimed the temperature was good for your body and you learned to accept it, even if your body was protesting with dizziness or nausea. During these years I sometimes felt awful during yoga, in a room filled with fifty people and without fresh air, with the temperature rising up to 120°F.

The rule at my studio, and at many others, was that you could not leave the room during the class because then "you won't be able to come back." I always proudly stayed in the room for the whole ninety minutes, no matter how terrible I felt. Moreover, you could bring a bottle of water in the room, but you could drink it only when the teachers allowed you, in the sequence after eagle pose. Looking back at this experience through the pillars of TCTSY, I am struck by the polarities. In the practice of Bikram there was directive language from the teacher and a total lack of control on the student's part, undermining any ability to *practice making choices*. If my body needed to rest or move at a different pace, I was expected to override this need and prioritize the expectations of the instructor over the wisdom of my body. I experienced invalidated *interoception*; for example, if I felt the need to drink, I was wrong because this is not the "correct" time to do it. Denying students the right to come and go as they please and punishing them should they leave the room are some ways that *coercion* showed up.

It seemed that most people doing the classes (including me) were feeling full of energy at the end. I now can reflect that I found this energy to be mostly negative, leading to aggressive behaviors. Luckily, the owner of the yoga studio had similar observations and decided to change style, moving slowly to a softer hot yoga, and started to lower the temperature weekly, ultimately reaching 88–90°F, a temperature that feels like a cuddle for my body, rather than the punishing heat of 104°F. The response to this change shined light on more of the problematic qualities with the practice of Bikram Yoga: Students at the studio became enraged about the temperature lowering, and some of them had aggressive behaviors toward the owner and the teachers. Approximately half of the numerous yogis attending the classes asked for a reimbursement and decided to change yoga studios. I saw people yelling at the teacher because of the lower temperature and slamming doors after the practice. This is an example of the impact that a teacher and culture in a yoga studio can have on us, and how easily the relationship between student and teacher can trigger past experiences.

After that, I tried different kinds of dynamic yoga: ashtanga, hot hatha, Forrest yoga, power yoga. I finally found Odaka yoga, which can be as physically intense as Bikram but softer in the teaching, using invitational language, shared experience, and choices. I finally felt that was the right practice for me. I felt more quiet—free to listen to my body and make choices. I began to explore making the choice to *not* push past my limits, which was a completely new concept for me. I felt more centered, more able to be in the present.

In the meantime, things were moving along in my professional life. I was working as a psychotherapist specializing in trauma and the treatments of eating disorders. In 2013 I co-founded a nonprofit organization for the prevention of eating disorders called Nutrimente Onlus, which in Italian means "nurture your mind." In 2015 a yoga teacher who practiced at my home studio proposed that we introduce yoga to folks we serve at my organization—usually clients already diagnosed with eating disorders or parents of teenagers starting to struggle with body image—or people who wanted to explore connection to their bodies.

Even though I wasn't a yoga teacher yet, I supported the group of yoga teachers and mental health providers in developing their approach for our clients. I did research on yoga in therapy, looking for published articles about yoga, eating disorders, and trauma, which is where I first learned about TCTSY.

During the first two years, I assisted with the sessions by participating and working with the yoga teacher to integrate some of what I was learning from the available books about TCTSY. We also worked to bring in the components of accessible yoga through a teacher who was trained as an accessible yoga ambassador. Accessible yoga has the mission to make yoga more available to all kind of bodies, offering adaptation of the postures, breathing, and meditation that meets individual body sizes and abilities, also with the creative use of props. What we created was an integration of trauma-informed yoga and accessible yoga. Clients we work with have a wide range of body types. We often utilized the accessible yoga approach to create a practice that was available to all bodies.

During these beginning years when we started to bring yoga to our clients, I began to understand that I needed more training in trauma-sensitive yoga. I had so many questions, and I wanted a deeper understanding of *why* I was finding yoga so effective. Doing clinical work requires that we trust our intuition, but the researcher in me knows that my intuition also needs questioning and scrutinizing. I wanted more data and knowledge to deepen my understanding of treating trauma through yoga.

When I finally did the training, I brought a lot of observations from my work that helped me understand the importance of the TCTSY pillars. In these first two years before formal training, we had teachers who had been trained to touch their students in order to adjust their postures. We found that for some clients it appeared to be useful, while for others anytime the teacher was coming to help and "correct," something in their face communicated that it was not okay or safe. After the teacher told a particular client, Anna, to sit on a block because her back was "too rounded" while sitting in a cross-legged form, Anna shut off and wasn't present at all during the rest of the class. But most clients described having positive impacts from the yoga sessions, like improvement in social abilities, more motivation in therapy, and a self-reported improved perception of their body. We also observed what Carolyn Costin and Joe Kelly describe in their book about yoga and eating disorders: the fact that clients finally felt that the body was *their* body.[1]

After receiving more training and becoming a facilitator, I started to offer TCTSY to both adult and teen clients with eating disorders. The power of the pillars became clear as I integrated them into my classes.

One of the profound impacts of eating disorders is the relationship to a body that is never thin, beautiful, or efficient enough. The relationship and connection to the body can be a significant barrier in healing, as it can be experienced as something "out of control" or unwieldy, and taking control of food is one of the most efficient (even if problematic) ways to feel less powerless. The exposure of your body in the context of a yoga class, where people can see you and you are invited to connect with your body, can be very challenging. As well, eating disorders very often involve some powerful beliefs and fears about the self that can make a yoga session very frightening—perfectionism (*I MUST be perfect*), absolutist thinking (*There is a right and wrong way to do things*), and the idea that making a mistake is catastrophic. In my opinion, these fears need to be addressed with more care when working with clients with eating disorders, and some TCTSY pillars are particularly important.

First of all, *choices* are crucial. Many clients with eating disorders have a high symptom severity and very long duration of illness, with onset at a very early age. During their lives the possibility to make choices is often very limited through being observed and judged. It is common for providers and family members to focus on what exactly clients are eating, how much they can walk or exercise, and when they are doing too much or too little of either. This means that, in addition to previous traumas that may have contributed to the cause of the disorder, clients are exposed to further relational trauma and power imbalances. This can lead to the experience of *I am not able to make any right choices for myself.* Moreover, clients with eating disorders often present some consuming thoughts and behaviors; for example, they might measure their belly to confirm it isn't bigger than the day before, eat food with the same colors, or wash their hands several times more than usual per day. When clients have experiences in treatment that undermine their sense of being able to make "good" or "safe" choices for themselves, even an A/B choice—for example, extending your arms overhead or leaving them at your sides—can be quite overwhelming. After

offering choice about how they might move, I found it very important to say: "If you prefer to not make a choice, you can do what
I'm doing, or do nothing at all." I understood that for some clients
it is very important to feel that they are supported in deciding to
follow me, doing their own thing, or choosing nothing. It became
clear that choosing to not move or participate is also a powerfully
important choice.

Another change that seemed to help the clients was having
the facilitator keep their eyes closed or looking down, rather than
looking around to "correct" clients. We also found that using the
names, like Warrior 1 or Tree, would send clients online looking
for the correct or perfect way to do the form, rather than building
trust in discovering how their body wanted to do the form. Some
clients would ask things like *Is this the fullest expression of the posture?*
or feel extremely inadequate if they couldn't do exactly what the
yoga teacher did. For clients who were constantly challenged to
let go of perfectionism, we ultimately found that not naming the
shapes allowed for a more present, sensory-based experience.

This thread of perfectionism showed up in other ways, as well.
In TCTSY we cultivate a shared authentic experience, which asks
the facilitator to explore their own interoceptive experience. This
also means sharing sensations they may be having, to serve as guideposts for participants. But the facilitator must consider how their
embodiment of the forms will impact those around them. For
example, I am very flexible, and many people are led to believe that
they should be flexible in order to practice yoga. Luckily, one of
my clients, with whom I have a very good therapeutic alliance, was
present during one of my first yoga classes and later commented on
how "flexible and good" I was at yoga. This allowed me to understand that my practice was taking up too much space in the room
and not allowing for clients to tune in to their own experience.
This led me to a practice of exploring my own interoceptive experience through noticing sensation when I did smaller or more subtle
movements. This change allowed the focus to shift away from my
"performance" and gave participants the opportunity to tune in to

their own experience. For me, this felt like it deepened my relationship with my body.

The pillar of non-coercion was the most challenging, and something that I continue to explore in my work. As providers we consider yoga a very important part of the treatment and do "push" clients to come try at least one session. In essence, we do coerce them. I have many conflicting thoughts about this. Clients with eating disorders often have to stay in imbalanced power dynamics with families and doctors for their whole life, because of the potential life risk of the illness, and I didn't want to reenact these power dynamics. But following that coercive start, I focused on giving them as much power as possible during the sessions, including using the Yoga Deck (yoga cards with different forms on them that the clients can choose). My dilemma was: if we don't push them, the risk is that they won't even try; but if we push them too much, we take away their power, just like they have usually experienced. So how can you nudge them to try TCTSY without forcing? In my experience it is not black and white, but what I tried to do is focus my language on sharing the power during the first classes; I also explicitly give them the choice to leave the class at any moment and come back only if they want to.

The pillar of interoception, in my experience, is the most important for clients with an eating disorder. Decreased interoception is considered to be a significant part of eating disorders, especially regarding the inability to recognize hunger or fullness. Very often such clients don't feel when their stomach is full and continue to eat until they feel pain, while in other situations they use behaviors to cover the sense of hunger, like chewing gum or drinking several coffees a day. There is disagreement in the field regarding the etiology of decreased interoception in clients with eating disorders. One hypothesis is that there is difficulty in making meaning of sensations in the body; another is that on a higher prefrontal cortex level, there is a nonacceptance of the internal experience.

The lack of interoceptive awareness in eating disorders has been proposed as a core symptom by psychiatry professor Hilde

Bruch.[2] The absence of the ability to recognize and define one's own emotions has been found often in anorexia nervosa, and it is believed to be one of the causes and reinforcing factors. Research has supported the generic assertion that women are less aware of their bodily sensations; this is especially the case in women who feel ashamed of their bodies and therefore deprive themselves by ignoring hunger and all the other internal cues, according to Katherine Dittmann and Marjorie Freedman.[3]

Moreover, inviting interoception in clients who have eating disorders often leads to a reduction of symptoms. Nayla Kouhry and colleagues gave an interesting meta-analysis on the effect of interoceptive improvements in different psychological and psychiatry illness.[4] It should also be noted that there are inconsistent findings in regards to eating disorders and interoceptive awareness. Sena Bleumel and colleagues found that the sensation of gastric satiation was higher in patients with anorexia, while in patients with bulimia stomach sensitivity was decreased. This reflects the heterogeneity of eating disorders and their manifestations—for example, food control, as in anorexia, and emotional eating, as in bulimia.[5]

Because of the hypothesized lack of interoceptive awareness in clients with eating disorders, the TCTSY facilitator needs to be very aware of the "dose" of interoceptive cues in a session. When I started to offer TCTSY sessions to teenagers with eating disorders, I decided to start with a low dose of interoception. During the whole session I gave only three cues to notice sensation within the body. When working with interoception I referenced a part of the body that typically has less emotional valiance, such as shoulders and neck, and avoided area that implicate a judgment, such as thighs, abdomen, or arms. Nevertheless, it was too much. The clients reported to their therapists that they were overwhelmed by the connection with their bodies, even if the cues to notice their bodies were infrequent and specific to certain movements. As a result of this feedback I found that the teens could tolerate introducing awareness of the body starting only with hands and feet for several sessions, before adding some cues about other parts of the body.

Adult clients were able to tolerate higher doses of interoception. They self-reported the ability to stay in their body, at least during the practice, and reported improvement in three to four sessions. They gave us feedback that after the yoga practice they could access the sensation in their bodies, recognizing the experience of thirst or fatigue. Almost all the adult clients kept their eyes open during the first one or two sessions but started to close them after the second one, while teens struggled in closing their eyes for several sessions. Most of them kept their eyes open widely, looking at me the whole session, signaling a barrier in turning toward internal sensation. In TCTSY keeping your eyes open or closed is always a choice, but when a client can feel safe in closing their eyes, it is a good sign of connection with the self. In the first few sessions we did a very brief resting pose for two minutes, but the adult participants asked to do it for more time. We tried introducing a very gentle body scan during resting pose, and it was definitely appreciated. At the end of the ten sessions, we were able to do a ten-minute resting pose with a body scan. Many clients shared this to be their favorite part of the session. The teens, in contrast, wanted a silent resting form, far away from the instructor. Building in opportunities for our clients to express what they needed—and then for us as providers to respond—was a central point in making the sessions safe.

There was also a paradox around interoception for many of our clients. The loss of interoception had a profound impact on them, and bringing it online seemed to have great benefits. At the same time, feeling sensation within the body was a completely new experience, and often very triggering. I had a powerful experience of noticing breath with one client. As soon as she noticed her breath, she experienced overwhelming anguish from the sensation of her abdomen moving. Another client had a panic attack during a balance form when she felt her leg shaking, which reminded her of a crisis when she was an inpatient. Although I have found interoception to be the most impactful part of the work with eating disorders, it can also be a liability. Facilitators need to be extremely careful, starting slowly and increasing interoceptive cues after learning more about the client's relationship and experience of feeling, and being aware of, their own body. Moreover, I would strongly advise being careful about the body area involved in interoception, as some areas that often have a cultural focus—such as thighs, abdomen, sometimes also arms—are quite vulnerable and can be deeply triggering.

                              §   §   §

Anna, a fifty-five-year-old woman and mother of four children, came to the trauma-sensitive yoga class on a suggestion from her therapist. She was working with her therapist on her attachment trauma. Anna had a very long history of psychiatric care, both outpatient and inpatient. She had three suicide attempts in the past five years, but her most profound symptom was binge eating. Whenever a painful emotion came up, she would find herself eating everything she could find in her kitchen very fast. Anna shared that because she had four children at home, there was often a lot of food in the house, making triggers everywhere.

Anna had tried hatha yoga during her most recent hospitalization, which resulted from a suicide attempt, and she found it useful as a way to connect to her body. She decided with her therapist that specific work on interoception and choice could be very useful for her. When I asked if I could write a clinical case on her, she was very happy to share her story; the narrative about her life, after one year of work on attachment trauma with EMDR, was very fluid. For a therapist working with trauma, a fluid narrative is a good sign that at least some part of the trauma is moving from being trapped in the body into conscious awareness so it can become speakable.

Anna didn't have many memories of her early childhood years, but her aunt filled in the details; Anna learned that after she turned one, her mother would beat her when she didn't eat. Her mother was also very critical of Anna, who would be verbally assaulted if she made a mistake like spilling something on the floor.

She started to think that something was wrong with her when she was ten years old, because what she did was never enough to please her mother. At the time she was doing artistic gymnastics, and her mother expected her to be a champion. As is often true, Anna didn't meet her mother's expectations. Any time Anna didn't medal at competition her mother insulted her, telling Anna she was a "weak person" and that she "disgusted" her mother. Anna's father didn't intervene or protect her, despite being present for this belittling. Anna expressed not enjoying competing, but she felt compelled to do it in order to please her mother, who was never satisfied with her performance even when she did medal. Anna was very good at school and liked to read, but that wasn't important to her mother, who continuously invalidated her preferences to read and study.

Anna started to overeat when she was fifteen years old, trying to find a way to manage her negative emotions, what she describes as her anger and sense of being "wrong." When she finished high school she thought that she was "not good enough" to go to university and stopped studying. Speaking with her, I could understand how many cognitive resources she has, and it was clear that if she had she gone to university she would have done very well. Her mother's disappointment continued to follow her. When Anna got married, her mother expressed her disapproval by coming to her wedding wearing black in mourning. Her mother never gave support, even when Anna asked her to go see a psychologist or when Anna had to stay in bed during her third pregnancy. As an adult she had to manage her mother's aggressive and passive-aggressive behavior. She decided to set boundaries in the relationship after her mother painfully rejected her when she asked for help preparing a Christmas dinner because she had three young children and expected a large crowd. After that moment, her mother cut off any type of relationship, as punishment for asserting boundaries, and she didn't tell her when her father became gravely ill. Anna was only able to see him the day he died.

After several years of different psychotherapies and hospital-izations, she came to work on attachment trauma in 2016, and to TCTSY in 2018. At the first session she appeared very anxious about exposing her body, which she considered much too big compared to others', because, as she told me, she was absolutely disconnected from her body.

In the beginning she shared with me that she had a hard time making choices and preferred to copy my movements. I reminded her that this is also a choice, to follow me. After the third session I saw her making more choices for her own body. Anna later told me she didn't like to sit cross-legged as all the other participants were doing, so she started to extend her legs on the floor. She could not close her eyes until the fourth session, and any time prior if I briefly looked toward her she was staring at me with her eyes open. During a TCTSY session, keeping eyes open or closed is always a choice; when a person feels that they can close them, it can be an indica-tion of trust and that they are feeling safe. Sometimes she asked me if she was doing it right; but I noticed that after navigating together how we don't have right or wrong forms in this practice but only the forms that felt okay for her in that moment, she soon under-stood that she could stop worrying about her performance.

After working together for quite a while, she told me that trying to do movements and forms, knowing that she would not be judged, was a completely new experience for her. "It made me discover a different angle of living with challenges that are inherent in my daily life. This empathic practice was useful to get inside myself, as if finding the best for me in that moment was not just a possibility, but a conscious choice of how I felt there and now."

During the course of the practices, which she continued weekly for nine months while continuing her EMDR (eye movement desensitization and reprocessing) psychotherapy, she reported an increased ability to perceive her body; this helped her reduce the binge eating and changed her relationship with food through the consciousness of what kind of food (and how much) could be healthy for her in the present moment. "Listening to the body is a way to learn to listen to yourself. To learn to be able to choose, in times of crisis, like when you have an uncontrollable desire to eat everything you have available, if and how you could act differently."

The experience of facilitating TCTSY was very useful for me, in both personal and professional ways. As a person struggling with her body, I found that yoga in general helped me a lot in accepting it and learning to understand my sensations—for example, knowing which kind of muscle I need to stretch if I feel some pain or stiffness in my neck. TCTSY moreover taught me how important it is to do yoga without the pressure of perfecting postures or striving for a goal; this means that you are centered and you *are* your body.

As a psychotherapist I clearly understood how TCTSY can be useful as an integrated therapy with eating disorder clients, but in my opinion sessions should be conducted by a facilitator with a deep expertise in working with eating disorders. They need to be aware of the most vulnerable parts of this disease, and they must adapt the sessions by tapping into this knowledge and being mindful of the effects of words, actions, and choices on this kind of client.

I would like to thank all the clients participating in my sessions for having taught me how the talk therapy we were doing was incomplete. I have learned that recovery cannot happen without supporting them in knowing and feeling that their body is *theirs.*

TAKING
EFFECTIVE ACTION

Be Myself; Be in My Self

OCD and My Movement toward Whole-Body Identity

Eviva Kahne

You are never stronger . . . than when you land on the opposite side of despair.

—ZADIE SMITH, *WHITE TEETH*[1]

THREE SUMMERS AGO, I LEFT a rooftop party and made immediate plans to fly across the world to come home.

The weeks before the flight, my body mind was out of control. I could not stop thinking about the idea of killing myself. My mind jostled. I desperately tried to force my thoughts into submission. I had filled up a notebook with reasons why I should not kill myself. I could not get this question out of my head. I had no idea why this thought was here or how to make it go away. I was cold at the thought.

A couple days before the flight, I sat in a dark hallway of an upper floor of the language school at midnight. I revealed a maddening truth to my father. I told him that in one way, the thought was preferable. During those tortuous internal moments, I was able to breathe.

These deep breaths were luxurious. I started having difficulty breathing six months prior, during my sophomore year of college. I remember the desperation at wanting to breathe: to fall asleep on the bus home from the science museum, to stop yawning as I worked at the writing center, to stop coughing during a DarkMatter poetry performance. These coughs and yawns made it so hard to be in my body, to feel okay. At the end of sophomore year, on the flight home before heading to Germany, I had a panic attack on the plane and felt somewhat unable to breathe for the nearly two-hour trip. As terrible as the thoughts were, I told my father, at least I could breathe.

In truth, the failed attempts to restrict and control—to regulate—both the thoughts and breaths brought despair. I felt fragile in my body: unsteady, empty, and distraught. I was completely uncertain of what was going on or how it would end or what would come after. I held onto this prose from *White Teeth*, with its offer of something existing beyond this despair.

§   §   §

I arrived in Boston, and my sister drove us to our family's cabin.

My sister was aware of my distress. She came prepared. She brought watercolors—we never used them. She and I made vegetable spring rolls and brownies. I had no appetite. I laid down on the couch, looked at crushes on Facebook, and read Cheryl Strayed's prose. I tried desperately to distract myself from my body mind. My sister took us to the side of the highway, and we picked wildflowers. Growing up I was constantly seeking my sister's attention and affection. She and I both desperately wanted me to be okay, and I wasn't. I was distraught in this patch of wildflowers.

That night, she held my body in our parents' bed. My mind was a storm. What the FUCK was going on? I felt so scared in my body. I remember this as a deep, fiery orange and yellow. I couldn't sleep. I couldn't lie still. I crawled to her on the second floor, upended. I pleaded with her: what am I gonna go? She said, you're gonna see someone. I said, they won't help. It's internal. How could they help control my own thoughts? She said, pleading back to me, I don't know. But even though I can't help and you can't solve it, there are people who can.

It was from this place—the place on my knees, the place of despair—that I came to yoga. But before I got to yoga, I drove with my sister back to Boston.

I stayed with her for a week and visited a therapist who engaged me in CBT: cognitive behavioral therapy. I was sent home with worksheets. The goal of these worksheets was to interrupt thought patterns, as a way to stop the uncontrollable thoughts causing so much suffering.

Something about this treatment did not resonate with me. All I'd wanted in those fiery weeks in Berlin was to control my thoughts, but controlling the thoughts did not feel like healing. I had two sessions with this therapist, and my relationship with CBT ended. It is miraculous that in the midst of so much suffering, my body could recognize that this treatment was not for me, was not serving my needs and deep desire to heal.

During that week in Boston, I spent all day lying on my back, while my parents figured out what to do. I waited until I could get a ride to go to the gym. I ran until I was so sweaty. On the treadmill, the thoughts were scary, and they did not stop me from running. And I was breathing. After running I would take a shower, go to the sauna, and lotion my body. In those daily three hours at the gym, I was in my body. This was my first experience with exercise, and with embodied healing.

That week in Boston, I stayed with my sister, and my dad took me to therapy and to the gym. Eventually he had to fly home for work. My sister also had to work. I remember sitting on the pavement outside a thrift shop, on the phone with my dad. No one knew what to do, where I should go. I decided to come home.

I got to Houston. I sat in my childhood home, on the couch, and filled out a questionnaire in preparation for a new therapist. I desperately wanted her to understand the turmoil inside my head. I wrote out all of my thoughts. I worked to be as comprehensive as possible, to let her into my mind and all its cycles.

When we met, we clicked. She got it. She saw me. She understood that the thoughts were unable to leave, that the thoughts

produced fear that prohibited me from trusting my body. She gave
me no worksheets. I said, I'm willing to work as hard as possible.
What should I do? What should I read? She mentioned a book on
acceptance and commitment therapy. Against my will, she gave me
no assignments. We talked for a few sessions. She told me about a
weekly class she held: a trauma-informed yoga class. I showed up
the following Wednesday.

The attendance was small. There was no socializing. There were
no assists. Over and over, I heard the refrain of the teacher: Pay
attention to the sensations in your body. You are never stuck in one
position. The message reverberating in my body was: Be present.
Be here, in my body.

Show up as Eviva, in a body, as a body, in full respect and attunement and presence. During theatre and in the first two years of
college, I was consumed by what it meant to be Eviva. Was she an
actor? A good enough actor? A good actor? Was she pretty enough
for boys? Was she smart enough for literature classes? What was her
major? Yoga was the first place where being Eviva was rooted in my
body. Showing up as Eviva meant showing up in my body. Recognizing the heat in my upper thigh during warrior 1, taking conscious
inhales and exhales with each pose. Taking care of my body was
showing up as Eviva.

In this period of practicing yoga, I had no structure for my life.
I was not in school. I was not working. I had left a study abroad
program with no major. I was healing because I had to. My days
consisted of going to therapy, yoga, and the gym. In therapy I
learned that the thoughts were connected to OCD, or obsessive-
compulsive disorder. I learned about the deep ties between OCD
and uncertainty.

The times I ran around Berlin streets and scribbling in my notebook, calling my sister, grandfather, mother: these times were a desperate attempt to stop the thoughts about suicide. The impulse to stop the

thoughts and find certainty in what these thoughts meant produced
so much suffering. Yoga encouraged me to be aware of my thoughts—
and at the same time, to be grounded in my full body mind.

> *Body-mind . . . recognize[s] both the inextricable relationships*
> *between our bodies and our minds and the ways in which the ideology*
> *of cure operates as if the two are distinct—the mind superior to the*
> *body, the mind defining personhood, the mind separating humans*
> *from non-humans.*
>
> —Eli Claire, disability justice activist and writer[2]

Healing happens in uncertainty. Healing comes from speaking
the thought, moving with the thought, and holding the thought:
not controlling the thought. The most revolutionary thing I have
ever experienced or witnessed was this paradigm shift of showing
up with my thoughts and in my body. Engage the pain, sit with the
suffering, acknowledge the sensation, pay attention.

When I practiced yoga in these early months of recovery, I was living
proof to myself that I did not need to have a plan for my life when I was
dedicated to healing and showing up for myself. This is a complicated
concept. I write nearly four years later with financial, work, and future
responsibilities that feel both easier and more necessary to gravitate
toward. When I get overwhelmed with responsibilities, desires, and
goals I want to manifest, it is powerful to reflect back on this time of
initial healing. The memories ground me. They point the way back
toward internal healing and restoration through exercise, yoga, meditation, and cooking. Internal healing did not come through certainty.
The desire for certainty created suffering. Internal healing came from
embracing uncertainty and showing up in my body.

Yoga also provided external as well as internal healing. I biked
to studios in my neighborhood and took Lyfts to studios downtown
and midtown. I used the communal showers, listened to the teachers,
and made friends with the front desk attendant. I was not alone in
the studio. My mat was one of five or fifty others. We were all witnessing each other, practicing this healing. Most of the time I witness
people on their phones. In yoga I witness people showing up for

themselves. That is nothing short of revolutionary. We were a care collective, not trying to fix anyone but to show up for ourselves, in ourselves, engaging the present moment.

§   §   §

In the year leading up to practicing yoga, my body and my relationship to my body were both changing. I met L. She was beautiful. Our compatibility blurred what I wanted from friendship and romance. My body danced with delight around her. I felt home.

As I engaged in yoga, my body engaged in other ways. During one class, I felt what I could only describe to my therapist as sexual energy. I had never articulated or felt that kind of heat before. I was on a mat on the far-left side of the room. There was music playing. My body was burning. There were sweaty bodies moving around me. I felt energy humming around my body as I flowed through the positions. It felt good.

Before the yogic awareness and sexual energy, I had experienced another new bodily sensation: back pain. A few days before leaving for Berlin, my back went out. I laid on the floor all day. My mother helped me onto the toilet. It was the first time my desire to stand did not manifest in my ability to do so. I was, for the first time, unable to move, with no knowledge of why it was happening or certainty about a resolution.

Just as a holistic relationship to my body was changing, so too was a relationship to my mind. No more worksheets. We engaged in a holistic therapeutic process, with elements of psychoanalysis. We talked about how I was feeling, about my familial relationships, about my fears and hopes for the future. What I don't remember talking about is high school theatre. The trauma.

§   §   §

Listening to *Dear Evan Hansen* lyrics out of context really frames my experience of high school theatre. From the song "Requiem," he was the flood, the fire, and the blaze.[3] The theatre teacher, the star, the blaze. He came from Broadway and Tony awards and New York. He blazed so bright that to be in his presence, I thought I shined too. He sucked up our love and work and talent like a vortex. More, more, more, laughed the Monster. Until I had nothing left to give. And still I did not walk away.

Let me tell you about the experience of being in the theatre department. Seven years after graduating, M, a friend whose friendship was torn in the vortex and rebuilt six years later, said to me: he capitalized on our immense need for belonging. That's the truth. From freshman year, to when he said, I'll make a star of you in senior year. My body shined bright with the potential of being powerful. Sophomore year, yelling No Ma'am, No More. I felt tiny, I felt like a fuck-up, the misfit in this theatre community. Junior year, I got a post-rehearsal note that said, "You were on fire." Somehow, that success belonged to him, and his stellar teaching, and not to me. And then, of course, the ultimate: senior year.

Instead of gearing up to leave high school, I was neck-deep in the vortex of this theatre space. I was president of our theatre troupe and one of the title characters in our spring show. I have select, horrific memories of this experience.

I am standing in front of the stage when the Monster tells me that I am not good as an actor. He recommends I go into outreach or theatre administration, that my energy and love of theatre will be well-needed there. I remember being threatened that if I did not get better in the role, I would get replaced. I remember feeling the darkness onstage. Once, my acting partner and I were locked in the Monster's office. He told us that the show was suffering because our relationship was bad. He said, fix it. My former friend said to me, you can't force a friendship. How do you respond to that?

Seven springs ago, right before our first competition. I remember the twelve-hour boot camps in a church open space. We all, including the teacher, spent the night in the church. I remember I couldn't sleep in the same open room as him. I was lying under a table. I could see him laughing with his friends, the sophomores who were better actors than I. Finally he fell asleep. My stomach churned looking at his closed eyes. I went to an adjacent small room and slept with another "not good actor."

In the mornings during the rehearsal process, I would imagine winning best actor at state. I needed so badly to be seen by others as great. All of my friendships and my entire identity seemed to depend on it: the school, my teachers, and family seemed tied to it. I was president of the International Thespian Society at my school. In this way I was at the center. Like the role, this position felt so fragile. This identity could be snatched up, I could be obliterated if the Monster decided I was not good enough. I was, at the same time, proud to be so visible, and suffering in the struggle to feel good enough. This coexisting tension feels emblematic of being at the center of someone else's structure. I felt stuck in this contradiction, sucked into the vortex.

As with other oppressive experiences, we turned against each other. I saw everyone as competition. The other actors were prettier, wittier, had more natural talent. I remember seeing the title actor in the dressing room before state competition. I don't remember exactly what he said. Something like: I fucking hate this. All of this. He won best actor at the state competition. I wished I could be that good.

There are many alumni who do theatre. They go to school for it, live in Los Angeles, produce films, build sets. I feel a kinship with those who stopped, about having been taken so horribly in this art form that somehow we have community through a shared traumatic experience. Because people with talent stopped, it made me believe that I, at one point, also had talent. Before the trauma.

It was over, and it wasn't.

I remember lying on the floor in my sister's Los Angeles apartment the summer after graduation. There was some event in Houston honoring our senior show, our director, and that time. I remember thinking I had to be there. I should be there. I felt a horrible pressure to be present. I had already graduated. I was across the country. I was set to start college in a matter of weeks. Yet this pull to come back into the vortex, to be in the presence of people who I both hated and felt unable to leave, was deep. My sister was sitting on the bed: You don't need to go. You do not need to go. I do not want you to fly home early to go. You have graduated. You have no obligation to be there. And I do not like the theatre department. I do not like the director. I do not like the way you were treated there. Why would you go? You had such a terrible experience.

I sat on the floor and drafted an email about how to make it to the ceremony. I looked at flights to leave Los Angeles. Would it be okay if I was thirty minutes late: how would people respond? I was having a great time in Los Angeles. I was in the middle of this computer vortex of making plans and swirling doubts when a turning point was made manifest in the room. I actually do not remember what my sister said here. What I do know is that she spoke truth about the poisonous environment of theatre. She made it clear that I did not have to be there. She spoke a truth I never imagined or knew that I wanted or needed: that I was done. That moment held an immense power: I felt an opening of life outside this vortex. Leaving that theatre space meant turning toward something so new, a light so blinding, I had no idea what I was stepping into.

That night, the fierce love of my sister was made manifest in that small LA room. She held me in bed until the sun came up. As I have moved through my life, I've found that the intimacy and power I have felt with women, whether it is familial, platonic, romantic, or even sexual, is unparalleled in its tenderness, strength, and beauty.

The Monster took up so much negative male energy in my life. He was entirely in control of my sense of self and self-worth. Theatre is an embodied practice. It centers on breath and movement. The Monster's power took hold in my body.

I did not go to yoga to resolve or address the trauma of the theatre department; however, I am curious how trauma-sensitive yoga might have responded to the experiences I had during high school theatre.

$\diamondsuit \quad \diamondsuit \quad \diamondsuit$

When I entered college I wanted something different. My body did not want to make space for someone to have that much power over me again. I did not want to feel so powerless in my body. That loss of agency in body would not resurface until the nonconsensual assist, four years later.

> I walked out of my yoga class today. I felt a heaviness in my chest and discomfort in my body. I wonder if the teacher noticed—she came over to me and massaged my neck. I couldn't tell if she was hitting on me. My lower stomach churns at the thought and I get a lump in my throat. I was trying to figure out how to ask her to stop—when I opened my eyes to attempt to say something, she stopped. I left shortly after. The feelings of discomfort I got then and when recalling the moment are visceral and painful. I did not feel connected or soothed by her touch—it felt activating. —My Journal, Saturday, August 11, 2018

What can I remember? I can remember the day I walked out of class. Standing by the door facing the studio, my mat was on the left, toward the back. I can remember her at the base of my neck. I remember that my eyes were closed and her hands were on my neck. I can remember wanting her to stop but not being sure how to say it. The rest of the class was quiet. I remember not wanting to disturb them, to make a scene, to have anyone hear me. I can remember lying there, feeling her fingers on my neck, my eyes closed. Feeling my palms on the mat, wondering how to tell her to stop. I can remember picking up my mat, walking out of class, walking to the locker room, feeling the strangeness of leaving. I can remember being in the parking lot outside of the studio. I can remember the heat of the moment. I can remember telling my close friend that this happened. I remember her response: I love assists. I love when they massage my neck. I can remember wondering if she was hitting on me. I feel anger: How is that an assist? How is that helping me feel a posture? I don't feel a heat of strength. I feel a heat of discomfort. This was one of my first intimate experiences, the first intimate experience with a woman, the only time I ever wanted an intimate experience to stop, and the only time I felt unable to say so as it was happening.

This nonconsensual assist occurred during a period of major transition and uncertainty. I graduated college two months prior, in May 2018. I had no job, and my childhood house was destroyed by Hurricane Harvey. I decided to move to Boston to be close to my grandparents. I would figure everything out from there.

> *I'll never know, and neither will you, of the life you don't choose. We'll only know that whatever that sister life was, it was important and beautiful and not ours.*
>
> —Cheryl Strayed, Tiny Beautiful Things: Advice on Life and Love from Dear Sugar[4]

I cannot prove, nor do I want to, that a nonconsensual assist prompted my leaving yoga. It is more powerful to consider the circumstances in which that nonconsensual assist occurred, and the subsequent major life uncertainties that unfolded shortly after. It is powerful to observe how the nonconsensual assist precursed a year of no yoga practice.

From October 2018 to May 2019, I worked three food service jobs. The longest one lasted five months. I was a prep cook and baker in a neighborhood café. The pay was terrible. We got a free lunch there, unlimited lattes, and desserts. I began to notice my pants did not fit me anymore. I started to dislike being in my body. It felt big. Lumpy. Extra. Food provides a feeling of security. But yoga does too. Food creates security by filling up space, and yoga does it by creating space.

My body was getting bigger, and I began to feel alienated from it. My body was again changing in other ways. My back pain moved from a dialogue to a scream.

Summer of 2019, I experienced two back spasms, far worse in pain than the one from summer 2016, or the minor flare-ups in the years between. The first time, I felt a sharp pang in the bathroom. I was unable to stand up or sit down. I cobbled my way to the floor and crawled back to my room. The next morning, a friend dressed me in fresh clothes on the ground. She offered me a hot towel to clean my aching body. She braided my hair. The second time, one month later, I experienced the worst physical muscular pain of my life. I was back home in Houston. I tried to turn on my side, and my body felt trapped. I screamed as loud as I could, then I called my parents. I slept in the living room with my father for days.

Soon after that spasm, but still recovering on the ground, I accepted, with elation, a job offer back in Boston. Since moving back, I have made fulfilling friendships for the first time since college. I have actively explored my sexuality and been physically intimate and open with new people. I moved into a co-op. My life became full. In some ways, overfull. It was not full with food. It was full with lots of new people, new ideas, new spaces. It was full; however, there was a critical piece missing. I was secure because I had filled up space with activities and people that excited me. But I was still not creating space.

Shortly after returning, I went to a talk called "Out of Darkness: Reconsidering Touch and Power Dynamics in Yoga." I remember sitting on the floor, surrounded by female-presenting bodies. One of the teachers invited us to think about power in the studio, a room with mostly female bodies in the #metoo era. Talking points around lineage, increasing visible bodily strength, yogic idols, and teacher's pets coalesced. None of this was what yoga was to me. Yoga was about creating space in my body. It was about turning toward that which had produced so much turmoil for me: breath. On the far-right side of the panel there was a young person. She was the most ardent one pushing for trauma-informed yoga. She was the youngest and least slim person on the stage. I saw myself in her age, sensibility, and body. My body, as I conceptualized it, and constructed from years of media consumption of feminine shapes, was somewhere in between these slim shapes and her own.

I had a crush—her combined aesthetic and powerful words were attractive to me. I believe part of the pain of that nonconsensual assist was that it occurred when I was in very early moments of processing my queerness and attraction to women. Feeling attraction to a woman, and having that woman exercise power over me in such a vulnerable moment, was both repulsive and heartbreaking. Over a year later, watching this woman speak about the crucial importance of being sensitive to trauma and touch provided a restorative experience for me.

When I first started practicing yoga in recovery, I was exercising every day. I felt my body get slimmer, tighter, tougher. It was a delightful and freeing feeling. Noticing my enjoyment of exercise, recognizing that I could feel good in my body, and having a body acceptable to external and internal expectations of femininity: all of these sensations and effects were new for me. When I graduated college, my circumstances as well as my body changed. I was in a new city and didn't know anyone. My back started to go out with more frequency and intensity. My initial experience with trauma-sensitive yoga was in a slim body. Coming back to it in this body didn't seem like an option, until I saw her.

As I settled back into Boston, I began to see a physical therapist. The refrain: keep moving. Your body is scared. That makes sense. It has gone through multiple spasms, with greater frequency and intensity. If you don't move, you will get stiff. The stiffness will convince you not to move, and this vicious cycle will continue. If you can move, you should. He went even further to say that pain in movement, in exercising, was not necessarily a bad thing. I was shocked. I thought I was supposed to stop at the first feeling or thought of pain. This concept bears powerful resonance with therapy: face the pain. With yoga: face the sensations. Pain, in and of itself, is not an inherently bad thing. To avoid it may bring more pain and isolation than I was initially trying to avoid. In a rounded way, the realization that pain needn't prohibit me from engaging with my body brought me back to yoga.

Today I practice yoga using YogaGlo. YogaGlo is an online app. I am not in the presence of any teachers. I have not yet had a chance to use a chip in a classroom. Since the nonconsensual assist, my presence in yoga studios has significantly decreased. In the YogaGlo app, I mostly, but not always, choose classes by women. YogaGlo provides a powerful way for me to engage in trauma-sensitive yoga. I know no one will touch me. I know no one will talk to me. Healing in yoga is both individual and collective. It is individual in that I show up in my body, observe, and respond to the sensations. When I use YogaGlo, the collective healing of yoga is not experienced. I have not experienced yoga in community, as a site of belonging.

I think what hurt the most from the nonconsensual assist was the recognition that yoga, space of healing and connection with my body when I began treatment, included an experience that violated my personal boundaries and made me uncomfortable in my body. It also happened by a woman. I was so used to feeling small by men. It was heartbreaking that this repulsive feeling could be activated by a woman.

So much of the trauma of theatre was about belonging. Everything I did in theatre was for him to love me. I dream that trauma-sensitive spaces will not only be confined to my headphones and bedroom. Yoga has allowed me to be in my body, to engage with my breath, with my bodily sensations, with my body on its own terms. I also want this healing to be public and collective. Feeling my power, being in my power, in the presence of others, is a powerful part of trauma recovery. Yoga, as an embodied practice, is inextricably tied to trauma.

Its focus on breath, movement, and awareness are deeply rooted in post-traumatic tendencies to avoid and control, and subsequently feel out of control. I want to experience this healing in community, where we are together, creating space for us to choose ourselves.

Yoga helps me want myself. So does eating nourishing food, meditating, journaling, hanging out with people, and working on projects where I expand. Yoga helps me expand. Instead of trying to be myself, I became aware of a practice to be in my self. Because the self is always changing—in sexuality and shape, in jobs and support network—it is much more important to me to feel rooted in my body than in an identity. Being rooted in my body holds space for me to feel all that I do and engage all that I am, always becoming.

I remember once, when I was home in early recovery, I reactivated my social media. My high school compliments page had tagged me in a post. The adjectives were very feminine-centric: "Eviva" is warm, fun, caring, wonderful. I remember one comment: her college is lucky to have her. High school theatre, questions of worthiness and being enough were stirred up by this comment, and who liked it. Sure, it made me feel good. All I'd wanted in high school was to feel loved and to belong. And yet something about this idealization of "Eviva" was deeply unsettling. I wanted out of that position, of always striving to be some unarticulated external and fixed idea of "Eviva."

The trauma of high school theatre still lives in my body, and so does the uncertainty of a year of underemployment and paralysis about next steps in my life. I subconsciously know that this lives out in my thoughts and decisions. What continues to live in my body is a tic disorder. Maybe it's not a tic disorder: medical diagnoses are powerful, at the least. My difficulty breathing remains in my body. It has changed over the years. In some places I notice its reduction. Other times its constant presence can bring frustration, exhaustion, and sadness. It has not brought despair.

Yoga has played a fundamental role in my relationship to my breath. Rather than trying to control my breath and feeling wildly out of control in that process, yoga encourages me to be with what is. Yoga is about paying attention to the sensations in my body. It involves bringing attention to my breath, which is so often a sight of anxiety for me. Yoga is about acknowledgment, about facing and engaging with what is. Yoga, to me, has always been trauma-sensitive.

My thoughts do not determine my identity. That was what terrified me in Berlin. External acceptance does not equal belonging. That's what I learned from theatre. My body is always changing. That's what I learned from back pain and size shifting. Through change, what stays constant is my body. I love the changes that have happened in my life.

In theatre I unapologetically and fervently believed that my self-worth and sense of self came from the approval of the Monster. After college I was convinced that having a job, any job somewhere in my interests, would reflect who I was. These are different circumstances; however, there is one threadline they do share. Both searched for external sources of identity. Most importantly, both require me to get chosen in order to be. With yoga, I choose me. Every time. The me does not depend on my thoughts or external approval, or even on my body form. It is an embodied me, in all its striving, anxieties, and uncertainties. It is whole.

Embers of Rage

Following the Sensations of Change

Anna Kharaz

AT THE CORE OF TRAUMA Center Trauma-Sensitive Yoga (TCTSY) is a deep respect for the importance of a process known as Reclaiming Your Body. In the aftermath of interpersonal and complex trauma, individuals can feel disconnected from, terrified of, or repulsed by their own body, which becomes the theatre in which the shadows of the past continue to play out. As a result, a critical aspect of healing from trauma is the process of reclaiming one's body, which occurs in three stages:

Stage 1: Having a body

Stage 2: Befriending your body

Stage 3: Using your body as a resource

For her doctoral dissertation in psychology, Jennifer West conducted a qualitative investigation of the impacts of TCTSY on women who have experienced trauma. In 2011 "Moving to Heal: Women's Experiences of Therapeutic Yoga after Complex Trauma" was published, and on page 46 she writes:

> The stage of "having a body" aims to heighten awareness of, and sense of ownership over, one's own body. As many survivors become disconnected from their bodily experience and/or view the body as out of one's control or "not mine," the "having a body" stage attempts to provide

a corrective and safe experience in the body and restore a sense of ownership. Once a person is able to feel comfortable and in control of her body, she can move to "befriending your body." This stage uses the awareness and ownership gained in the first stage to emphasize the notion of getting to know one's bodily experience and then choosing how to move in a way that feels good. From here, "body as a resource" allows for the building of skills for self-regulation (Emerson & Turner, 2010). In other words, students/clients begin to see their body as a tool to calm oneself down (e.g., through breathing or soothing movement).[1]

As a therapist and TCTSY facilitator, I've always felt this multistage concept of Reclaiming Your Body resonating with me as I've reflected on the complex reasons so many survivors are often deterred from practices that include their body, despite its potential for healing. I have come to believe that this may be an extension of the fact that many body-based practices, including yoga, are most often taught with the assumption that participants are in stage 2 or 3 of the Reclaiming Your Body process. This is a great disservice to those seeking healing who may not be able or ready to see their body as an inhabitable, safe, consistent, predictable, or welcoming place. Furthermore, showing up to do yoga with a teacher who loves, flaunts, and celebrates their own body could further shame and invalidate survivors and send the message that this practice is only for those who already love and accept their bodies.

Since incorporating TCTSY into my work as a clinical therapist, I have come to learn that the sequence of this process, much like trauma healing in general, can be nonlinear in nature. Someone can be in stage 2 one week, stage 1 the next, and stage 3 the week after. Our work as TCTSY facilitators, which requires careful attunement and a deep dedication to engaging in a non-coercive relationship, means meeting our participants wherever they are at any given moment. This might change week to week, session to session, and moment to moment. On rare occasion, someone might even cycle through these three stages in these same sixty-minute sessions, as happened one dreary Tuesday evening in September with Nicole.

Nicole is a twenty-five-year-old woman who originally sought therapy for the residual effects of a sexual assault her junior year of college. In the waiting area and the therapy office alike, Nicole takes up little space. She often sits as if she's purposefully trying to make herself more compact, holding her arms close to the sides of her body, her fingers tucked into the crease behind her knees. She comes to our sessions straight from work, always dressed modestly and professionally. Often between sentences she pauses to gather her thoughts, her left arm momentarily leaving the side of her body to delicately adjust her glasses. She seems to choose her words and movements carefully and always comes "prepared" with a topic of conversation for our sessions.

When we first met, Nicole told me that the assault itself wasn't even the worst part of the whole experience and that there were two exacerbating factors to her pain. The first was continuing to live on her college campus, always within a half-mile radius of her perpetrator. The thought of his physical proximity was always lurking in the backdrop of her mind, keeping her up at night and distracted all day. The second exacerbating factor was that, after she found the courage to reach out to her university's administration, the staff there failed to believe, listen to, or support her. Later when Nicole tried to share her experience of sexual assault with her parents, her mother instantly shut down, continuing the cascade of a pattern that has haunted Nicole since childhood: people who should be there to help and support instead fail and create more harm. Shortly thereafter Nicole learned that her mother was a survivor of sexual assault herself, at the hands of her own father (Nicole's grandfather).

Realizing the potential underlying reasons for Nicole's mother's inability to offer nurturance to any of her four daughters still has not made up for what Nicole has been missing her entire life. In fact, Nicole has shared with me that she only learned about "what mothers are supposed to do" by watching other moms' parenting: the moms who picked Nicole's classmates up from school or those who stood on the sidelines of Nicole's soccer games. Those were the moms who taught Nicole that something was missing, that something wasn't quite right. Sometimes when she thinks about the care, love, and support she never received, Nicole still feels a bottomless void in her being that can never be filled.

One day Nicole mentioned the irony that her favorite book growing up was *Are You My Mother?*, a lighthearted tale of a newly hatched bird in search for his mother. Nicole notices herself laughing as she tells me this, but shares that inside she feels "so sad for that little girl." She wipes the tears from her eyes, the laughter now gone. "I wish I could tell her that it won't always be this hard."

Like the hatchling in the book, Nicole has also spent much of her life in search of a mother figure. Having become accustomed to her mom being "a 'no' person," as Nicole calls her, she learned that seeking connection from her mother was a pointless quest. However, despite her father's conditional warmth and acceptance of his daughters, she discovered a loophole. Nicole's father grew up as the star athlete of whatever sport he played and continued his love of soccer by coaching local youth leagues in their small town. Nicole learned that she could get close to him by being the best at soccer . . . and so she did.

Nicole became the top player on every soccer team she played on. She put all her effort into becoming the best and watched her relationship with her father blossom and grow. Her training was physically challenging but socially grueling. Nicole once reflected that "to be a competitor in soccer, you couldn't really have friends. That wasn't what a competitor did. Competitors are cold, jerks, and generally relentless. Essentially everyone is competition." Her teammates, envious of her abilities, would find reasons to taunt and tease her on the field and then exclude her from their after-practice hangouts and weekend sleepovers. Nicole adjusted to a life of conditional connection with her father at the expense of relationships with her peers.

After Nicole suffered her fourth soccer-related concussion, her post-concussive syndrome became completely debilitating. The headaches, inconsistent concentration, word-finding difficulties, and memory loss made daily life excruciating—and playing soccer impossible and downright dangerous. Just like that, Nicole's identity and primary mode of connection became extinguished. When Nicole's future assailant, then nothing more than a friendly classmate, approached her for help on a shared homework assignment, Nicole gladly accepted. She was now desperate for connection and eagerly seized the opportunity to make a friend in the process. Later, after he sexually assaulted her, Nicole's sense of self, safety, and connection was only further depleted, leaving her stranded in a sea of betrayal, shame, and loneliness.

During Nicole's sexual assault she became frozen and submissive, a protective and brilliant sympathetic nervous system strategy that allowed her to survive the experience she faced. This same response, learned by her nervous system as a way to protect her from threat, took over whenever she was faced with an experience that reminded her of this original trauma.

After her assault, Nicole could feel a tremendous amount of rage, which had to be numbed in the presence of her assailant to keep a bad situation from becoming worse. In the months following her assault, it was this rage that empowered her to become an active university member, standing up against sexual violence and helping fellow classmates voice their stories and feel less alone in their experiences.

When she and I went through the symptoms of post-traumatic stress disorder early in our work together, Nicole expressed the tremendous relief she felt when she realized how many of the thoughts, feelings, and behaviors she experienced on a daily basis met the criteria of this condition. For the first time, she started to make sense to herself.

Back on that dreary Tuesday evening in September, Nicole enters my office uncharacteristically angry. We have been working together for about a year at this point, using a combination of TCTSY and talk therapy, and it's unusual to see her so activated. I learn that an interaction with a co-worker has left her enraged. Nicole describes how small and disrespected she felt as a large male co-worker stood looming over her, talking down to her, as she sat quietly, shrinking into her chair with his every word, frozen and unable to speak.

This work interaction, with its subtle and overt similarities to Nicole's past sexual trauma, activated her sympathetic nervous system, spiraling her into the implicit memory of that one night in college.

Now, in my office, Nicole's system returns to this sympathetic nervous system oscillation that ensured her survival during the original trauma. Brilliantly hijacked by the "fight" part of her that has learned to follow her "freeze" response, Nicole's rage is audible in her speech and visible in her tense body posture as she enters my office this particular day. Over the next sixty minutes, Nicole embarks on the journey of reclaiming her body and emerges a more embodied, regulated, and empowered version of herself.

Stage 1: Having a Body

As her anger builds, I validate the injustice of what ensued earlier that day and ask Nicole, "Would you like to keep talking about this situation, or would you like to move your body?"

"Yeah, I feel like I need to move actually," she says, the agitation surfacing in her normally calm and collected voice.

"Do you know how you'd like to move today, or would you like me to guide us through some movement?" I ask.

She chooses the latter, and I begin to guide us through some seated yoga movements: head circles, shoulder movements, and arm movements. As we do these shapes together I ask, "Do you notice anything in your body?"

She says, pensively, "I'm starting to feel heat in my hands and in my chest."

This is the moment Nicole shifts into stage 1 of the Reclaiming Your Body process. She showed up disconnected from her body, unable to notice its internal messages but consumed by its physiological implications. Now she becomes aware of its not-so-subtle language, emerging here in the sensation of heat, which she so eloquently was able to name (a feat in and of itself, given the nonverbal nature of trauma).

Stage 3: Using Your Body as a Resource

"Would you like to work with this sensation of heat in your hands and chest, or would you prefer to keep moving in the way we have been?"

She chooses the former, and we begin to explore these sensations. We try adding movement and pausing in stillness, all while keeping careful track of how they impact the sensations Nicole notices in her body. After a few minutes of exploration, Nicole finds that if she vigorously shakes her hands, she can feel the heat in her body dissipate. Nicole has now shifted from stage 1 into stage 3 of the Reclaiming Your Body process, realizing that she can change how she feels by moving in different ways. We continue to explore this, trying different kinds of movement together and seeing what feels useful and what does not. After a few more minutes of this, I ask Nicole if the heat in her body is still the same or if it's changed at all.

"The heat is gone but there are still embers in my belly. I'm thinking about the work thing again, and I feel like this feeling in my belly is saying 'my time is valuable' and 'I just want to be respected.'" As Nicole voices this realization, she notices the sensation in her belly subside, and she tells me she'd like to move to the ground so that she can do some physical therapy exercises for her knee, on which she recently underwent surgery for a torn anterior cruciate ligament (ACL). As the sensation of heat and embers dissipates in her body, she becomes aware of "a lot of tightness" and "discomfort" in her knee and notices she'd like to stretch it.

Stage 2: Befriending Your Body

Nicole now enters into stage 2 of the Reclaiming Your Body process, curious and motivated to ease the discomfort in her knee. She is now guiding our movement with her physical therapy exercises, and I follow along, mirroring her as she tells me about the soccer game she played this weekend, likely contributing to the feeling she has now in her knee. This was her first soccer game since her surgery, and she proudly tells me of the goal she scored in the first few minutes. Her voice, affect, and presentation are now different. She appears calmer and more present, and while she becomes more connected to her own body, I notice how this changes our relationship as well. I find myself more at ease in her presence and feel more connected to Nicole. I note this simply as information, that perhaps Nicole's nervous system has shifted out of a trauma response, back into the present moment.

Nicole's athletic ability has always been a tremendous source of pride to her, and now that the residual sensations of the workday's "embers" have quieted, she can reconnect with her internal strength, pride, and self-esteem. We stretch a while longer together, until Nicole notices that her knee is feeling much better and more flexible. She smirks and looks down at her knee, with a certain warmth in her gaze, and says, "Thanks for working so hard."

As she gently pats her recovering knee, we both get teary-eyed, moved by this tender moment of connecting with herself. The session soon comes to an end.

§   §   §

In looking back on this session, there were a few lessons that have been useful to me. Following the session, my initial reaction, upon recalling the concept and process of Reclaiming Your Body, was confusion regarding the sequence of events. How could Nicole have gone from stage 1 to stage 3 to stage 2? I felt the confusion arising in me soften when recalling the nonlinear nature of this work and the fluidity and uniqueness of this process for each individual.

This realization served as a useful reminder of the ways in which we, as providers, can veer off track because of our own agenda. Sometimes this agenda can include kind-hearted thoughts and well wishes such as *I wish for my clients to feel less anxious, so I will focus on this in my sessions.* Sometimes our agenda can include our own rigid belief systems, such as what I felt shortly after Nicole left my office: *The sequence of a process should be linear and chronological.* An agenda can also include the dangerous territory of responding to our own affective or somatic experiences, which can show up for therapists and yoga teachers alike.

As humans it is normal for us to have a physiological response (manifesting as sensation, affect, and cognition) when witnessing the emotional expression of another. Though this is a healthy process, it can create a ripple of harm if not carefully observed by the beholder.

When Nicole arrived at my office activated and noticeably distressed, I could feel my body react in the way it typically does around expressions of anger. My system has learned to go on the defense when faced with someone's rage: my heart rate increases, my hands perspire, my chest muscles constrict, and my breathing becomes shallow. If I weren't in tune to this reaction, I could easily fall into the trap of prescribing coping strategies to Nicole to help her regulate her anger so that I could feel more at ease in my own body during the session.

This act of subtle coercion, under the guise of modern talk therapy, would re-create the power dynamics inherent to interpersonal trauma: namely that I, as the therapist in this situation, am clearly in charge. To avoid mimicking the trauma paradigm, it is my responsibility to instead notice my reaction and manage it internally, without having to coerce Nicole into changing her emotional expression. This allows me to be able to better tolerate being present with Nicole's affective experiences.

Interestingly, Nicole later shared that the session described here was "probably the quickest I have ever processed/moved through something that triggered me."

The lesson for me was that, even though I didn't prescribe self-regulation strategies or remind Nicole to use her coping skills, she moved through the experience on her own and, through this place of empowerment, shifted her internal world. I have come to believe that it is only within this cocoon of non-coercion that the Reclaiming Your Body metamorphosis can take place.

For me, the brilliance of this framework is that it silences all the other noise in the room. All the distractions I can inadvertently hook into as a care provider become quieter when I remember that our primary goal in this work is to be present with whatever shows up in the moment, in the container of a relationship founded on non-coercion and empowerment. Through this process of reclaiming what should never have been taken away in the first place, the wisdom of the body can unfurl, and the past can slowly become a thing of the past.

Finding My Soul

A Team Approach to Healing

Dallas Adams, Kayla Marzolino, Sonia Roschelli, and Jessica Rohr

I first met Kayla on her second day on the inpatient unit. Kayla was well-coiffed, personable, and easy to talk to. She was clearly a people-person, and she had a sort of untouchable presence about her. Her treatment team enjoyed her, and it became quickly apparent that it might be tough for her to show vulnerability after years of practice in appearing strong. She had a significant trauma history with a lot of invalidation about that trauma, and she had been taught that her worth was in her appearance. She was bright and incisive, and she used what she learned about herself and the world to move within it very effectively; the major downside was that this involved her invalidating her own experience much of the time. This came up in therapy, when she described that even on the unit, when an older man said inappropriate things to her, her instinct was to keep the peace and ensure everyone's comfort rather than say something assertive back that might "ruin" everyone's moment. The choices she made served someone else's values—her abuser's, her mother's, society's. Working together, she quickly recognized that she actually knew very well what her own values were; she had just been out of practice with connecting with them. —Jessica, Kayla's individual therapist

Trauma Center Trauma-Sensitive Yoga (TCTSY) is an evidence-based yoga practice that specifically speaks to many of the difficulties patients with a complex trauma history have. To address the disconnect patients often feel between their mind and their body, TCTSY teaches interoception, or building awareness of their physical and emotional experience. This helps patients build healthy relationships with themselves and others. To address the sense many patients have that their choice was taken from them long ago, they are taught trauma-informed strategies such as choice-making and consistent opportunities to take effective action. According to Dave Emerson, co-founder of TCTSY, taking effective action involves "muscular dynamics which students purposefully initiate in order to make themselves feel more comfortable. The key is planning based on some experience and then acting, not just thinking about your plan."[1] Taking effective action in TCTSY applies to patients adjusting their bodies in the session in order to feel more comfortable; this can also apply to patients learning to move differently through their world in order to feel more comfortable with themselves, their bodies, and their relationships. For many people, the simple act of choosing a different action leads to a new and powerful sense of agency.

> I didn't know that I wasn't already empowered. I didn't realize that it was okay for me to do something slightly different. And one day, he did a pose, and I thought, "I'm not doing that, I'm doing something else." Then I was thinking, "Oh my gosh, I'm doing another pose. I'm not doing everything everyone else is doing." It gave me a sense of pride. It started helping me find my words again. Find my voice. Find my soul. —Kayla

TCTSY has been implemented since 2015 at The Menninger Clinic, a psychotherapeutic hospital in Houston. Menninger uses a team approach that identifies the patient as the most important member and includes other providers from multiple disciplines, including a psychiatrist, psychologist, social worker, nursing staff, mental health associates, psychosocial rehabilitation therapists, individual therapists, family therapists, and addiction counselors and eating disorder specialists as needed.

The patient's (and their family's, if desired) participation in treatment is essential to our model of recovery. We know that the more the patient is involved with us, their team, the better their results are in terms of their ability to achieve their goals. We believe this is beneficial in several ways. First, patient-centered care is trauma-informed, as patients are in control and have choice about treatment they participate in. Second, this level of participation, choice, and informed consent enhances the possibility of treatment adherence here and at home. Third, it emphasizes the importance of each patient taking agency or responsibility for their care and their well-being. Finally, while Menninger uses state-of-the-art treatment modalities and interventions, a key part of the culture and treatment here is the belief that the relationships patients develop with staff and each other through this team approach are often the most helpful and healing elements of treatment. Together these patient-led multidisciplinary teams identify and address the patient's core issues through comprehensive assessments, recommended evidence-based groups, family therapy, and individual therapy, as well as adjunctive and rehabilitative therapies over a period of four to eight weeks.

After completing treatment, many patients share that the relationships with one another were the most helpful component of their admission. This is important because we know that survivors of complex trauma can have disrupted relationships of all types, and the trauma may have physiologically, emotionally, mentally, and spiritually impacted their ability to successfully and confidently navigate their world over time.

I knew about TCTSY from hearing Dallas describe it in a meeting, but my understanding was purely academic. I understood that it was effective if a certain number of sessions were attended, and I was happy to hear about an evidence-based yoga practice available to our patients, but I didn't have a deeper understanding of the in-the-moment ways the intervention worked. I don't know that I had actually ever spoken about it with a patient before Kayla brought it up in our session. —Jessica

When implementing TCTSY, it is important for facilitators to do so as closely as possible to the recommendations made by the developers. At Menninger, members of the yoga group are determined by a referral from the patient's team. Treatment teams are regularly provided education on the criteria for membership. When orienting patients to the intervention, facilitators first ask whether the patient knew about the referral and what their understanding of TCTSY might be. The facilitator describes TCTSY as an intervention for people with complex trauma with the goal of increasing connection between brain and body, highlighting the neurological, trauma-theory, and relationship perspectives. They share that TCTSY increases awareness of sensation and provides opportunities to practice making choices about how patients use their body. Facilitators provide verbal cues for the forms to take, and they emphasize choice. Patients choose whether to do a different yoga form, how long to hold their form, and whether to engage in the poses at all. (On one occasion, a patient chose to take a nap!) The facilitators also encourage patients to take their experience back to their team and individual therapist to make meaning of it.

When I first got in the class, Dallas said, "This yoga has been shown to decrease the effects of trauma by 33 percent," and I thought, wow. If that's true, that's incredible. Then he got into the poses, and at first he was saying, "It's your body, you can do what you want." I thought, "I get it, I get the game. We're supposed to feel empowered, I get it." I went through it anyway, and it was still kind of enjoyable and peaceful, and I thought, "If these benefits are true, I'm sticking with it."

At one point, my social worker was trying to make my family therapy call during that time, and we had to explain that you have to have a certain number of sessions to be really effective. We reworked part of my schedule to allow me to stay in there. —Kayla

Patients are told about the NIH study for the effectiveness of TCTSY, where post-traumatic stress disorder symptoms were reduced by 33 percent after participants attended ten sessions.[2] They are asked to commit to attending each meeting both to receive benefit from the intervention and to help create a sense of safety in the room, as all group members feel safer when they know who will be in the room with them. If three sessions are missed, patients are not asked to return, and the patient's interdisciplinary team is expected to respect scheduling. This means that teams do not schedule other appointments during the group time and that staff remind patients as appropriate that they have choices to attend the group or not. Finally, they are reminded to work to process trauma and other experiences with their individual therapist and their team, as TCTSY is not the place for process work.

It is rare we hear about the experience patients have with TCTSY from other providers, and Sonia [TCTSY co-facilitator] and I found this to be rewarding, helpful, and encouraging. Not knowing patients' experience and history allows me to simply be in the room with them, offering them opportunities to notice sensation, make choices, stay in the moment, and take effective action if they choose. The difficult and freeing part of this means they get to choose how they wish to be in that time; what they experience is up to them. It means I have to trust they are doing the best they can for them at that time and that they are the experts about themselves. Essentially I am holding space for them and they are in control of their body. —Dallas, TCTSY facilitator

We bring a discussion of TCTSY as a component of treatment during a voluntary admission to The Menninger Clinic. Just as with the parable of blind men touching different parts of an elephant and labeling their experience differently ("It's a tree!" "It's a big snake!") based on their limited information, teams at a hospital can become siloed and find themselves fully immersed in their own experience and unable to integrate moments into a cohesive whole. We hope to show a glimpse of the different ways a simple ten-session course of TCTSY impacted a patient's treatment, her general recovery, the TCTSY practitioners themselves, and her individual therapy. The reader can imagine the ways that the lives of the practitioners and the patient paralleled, intersected, and diverged.

We'll begin with commentary from TCTSY facilitator Dallas.

Our experience in facilitating this group is fairly straightforward. Because this group occurred at the end of the workday, Sonia and I noted that we often feel tired and reluctant as the time for group approached. We also note, though, that as we begin to go to each unit and pick up group members to take them to the group room, this tiredness begins to dissipate. As the group progresses, we often feel more energized and glad to have persevered.

During the time Kayla was in the group, we were aware of particular difficulty with certain members tolerating transitions from one form to another. We were aware of ourselves feeling resentment about it and afraid it was distracting from others' experiences and what the implications of that might be. We discussed this experience with each other, and one of my worries was that other group members might find it so annoying they would quit coming to the group. Sonia and I really struggled to find how to best respond to this difficulty. Speaking directly to it by giving cues and more options in the group was one option. Another was to speak directly to the members having difficulty. Our fear was that these two choices would be ineffective and/or shame or alienate the patients. Instead we chose to slow the pace to one more manageable for the group as a whole, and this seemed successful in reducing the difficulty.

I was aware Kayla had to reschedule her family session with her husband and social worker so she could attend the groups regularly. I remember feeling impressed that she, her husband, and her social worker were on board with TCTSY intervention such that they were willing to adjust. Kayla attended nine sessions prior to discharge. She usually was located in the front of the room and occasionally experimented with forms that were different than what we expressed, which is consistent with the spirit of TCTSY. Kayla and I really did not speak with one another during her treatment, except when she was trying to reschedule her family therapy sessions. It was not until shortly before she left that Kayla's therapist, Jessica, reached out to me to let me know how helpful Kayla had found TCTSY.

This occurrence, as well as co-authoring this chapter with my colleagues and with Kayla, has been a really powerful learning experience for me. Part of my role as facilitator of a TCTSY group is to hold space for people to learn about themselves via experiencing sensation, practicing choice, and taking effective action. In both situations, I held space for and actively supported people learning about themselves. Patients were experiencing difficulty in transitioning from one form to another, and Kayla had found her own voice. When people then act on that knowledge—in these two cases by making their difficulty known and when Kayla actually began to share with us her perceptions about the relatability of the article to the identified audience—I had to incorporate those views. As I think about this, incorporating those views began to change the power dynamics, and I and the other patients and Kayla became much more partners in the processes, which created a new level of responsibility for them and for me, and to each other and to ourselves. This shift creates new anxieties for me that at one level are exciting and another can be frightening, and it creates some anxious feelings in my stomach and shoulders as I have less of the "all-knowing facilitator" facade to hide behind. I wonder if the . patients and Kayla experience similar sensations and feelings.

What is clear as I write this is that not knowing and whatever feelings come with that are my issue and not the patient's. When, as discussed earlier, group members risk asking for assistance and interacting, the question for me becomes how to continue to support their experience while also considering responding in a way that opens the possibility of more of a partnership between myself and the group member. This will clearly be a growth edge in the future for me, one that could not have occurred without these two powerful experiences.

Next we'll have commentary from TCTSY co-facilitator Sonia.

I began to shadow and help facilitate TCTSY with Dallas right after I had completed my 200-hour registered yoga teacher training. I spent time with Dallas learning about TCTSY from him as well as reading David Emerson's book. Coming out of training and brand-new to teaching, I had learned a certain way of leading a class in a practice, which involved being rather directive, offering physical assists, and correcting forms when students were not in them properly. I had been taught about anatomy and a certain philosophy of practicing yoga forms that resonated well with my body, and it made sense to me that it would also work well for others. I was quickly able to see the differences between TCTSY and the way I was taught to lead a class. The changes in the way the group was led in TCTSY made sense to me, given what I know about trauma, and it felt easy to go along with this change when I began co-facilitating.

As I learned more about Dallas and Kayla's internal experiences through the process of writing this chapter, I got in touch with my own parallel process—that is, my own similar experience that I was working through at the same time. Because our group at that time was experiencing difficulty in transitioning from form to form, I found myself wishing that Dallas or I would speak to it directly in the room, giving cues to the group as a whole, as a way of "correcting" it. I was hoping that through this we could gain some control back and effectively manage the anxiety and frustration that this issue left with me. As Dallas pointed out, this would likely have reinforced power dynamics of him and me as "know-it-all facilitators" instead of partners in a process. This collaboration increased my anxiety as it felt more vulnerable and out of our control. It required trust on all of our parts, patients and facilitators, with ourselves and each other.

Before this point, I logically understood why we facilitate TCTSY in a different way from a more traditional yoga class, but it was in this situation that I *felt* what it meant to collaboratively hold space for people in the group to discover experiencing sensation, practicing choice, and taking effective action for themselves. What I see as a problem to be corrected may be a part of someone else's learning process about themselves. Responding with control to relieve my anxiety (rather than managing it myself) robs the group of the opportunity to discover and take effective action for themselves. To let go of this control requires me to trust the process, myself, and the group. I began to notice how this experience in the TCTSY group paralleled my own yoga practice, where I often struggle with inversions (forms where my heart is higher than my head); I feel out of control and hesitate to trust myself in these forms because of worries that I will fall and what might happen as a result. It is only when I learn to let go of the control and trust the process that I can grow in my practice. This experience allowed me to see how this process plays out for me on and off of my mat, as well as find better ways of taking effective actions that work for me and allow space for exploration, discovery, and choice for myself and others.

※　※　※

We'll move on now to commentary from Kayla's individual therapist, Jessica.

Kayla came to therapy ready to work and aware of some of the more significant issues that had shaped her life; however, it took some work to identify how strong her patterns of protection had become after years of using them. This shield of beauty and wit that she used to keep a close handle on her interactions was effective in keeping her separate from her experience, which meant that she had moved further and further away from connecting with her emotions and her world.

As time went on, we worked together on her sense of her connection with the world; a topic that came up quite a bit was her sense that she was doing everything she was supposed to be doing— she married a great husband, had beautiful kids, was financially stable—but she still wasn't happy. This idea of "doing what she's supposed to do" pervaded therapy, and it wasn't until she had a major breakthrough in TCTSY that she began to explore and feel the joy and meaning of *not* doing what she was supposed to do, but doing what made sense and worked for her. This breakthrough for Kayla came after a few sessions of attending TCTSY with some hesitation and cynicism; as an intuitive and protective person, she quickly understood what the goal of TCTSY was and fell into old patterns of experiencing it from a distance. In one session, however, she caught herself being cynical and pushed herself to give up a little bit of control, which actually allowed her to feel even more ownership than she realized she could. It was a simple moment, when Dallas reminded the TCTSY attendees that although he was suggesting a pose, they were in charge of their bodies and could do whatever they wanted. Kayla heard this clearly for the first time, and she did exactly what her body told her to do. This was powerful for her, to be able to connect with her body and act with it in a way that was meaningful and important to her and her alone, and she experienced that as good and worthwhile. TCTSY seemed to be the place where she could explore that the most, while discussing and being curious about ways that she could start to change outside of yoga.

We discussed again her experience of hearing an inappropriate comment and her natural response, which was "keeping the peace" by making a dismissive remark that helped her not to engage but didn't provide the commenter with any feedback. We processed this for a while, exploring the idea of *not* keeping the peace in favor of leaning into her self-respect and what that might look like. TCTSY gave her the chance to practice not keeping the peace for the sake of someone else and doing things that made sense for herself and her body. There is also a tendency for people who develop insights into some of their patterns that may be interfering with their best life to start to denigrate or distance from themselves entirely; for example, a person who has difficulty with strong emotions begins to completely ignore emotions in order to try and "recover." Kayla was aware of this tendency and retained the parts of herself she loved; she continues to be well-coiffed, incisive, witty, and kind. She also is learning how to show that love for herself by owning her space and empowering her body, and this was reflected in her love for TCTSY and her decision to continue studying as a yoga teacher to bring that love to other people.

I was thrilled to work to incorporate her experience in TCTSY into our work. There is almost nothing more effective than in vivo (or real-life) experiences to help build awareness and practice exposure to discomfort. For her to have the opportunity to do something her body felt good doing and her mind felt safe exploring was just wonderful.

Finally, let's hear from Kayla regarding her experience. Jessica, Dallas, and Sonia talked with Kayla for this piece, and they've left it in interview format to maintain the integrity and flow. It has been edited slightly to protect patient information and improve readability.

Jessica: *How did you first learn about trauma-sensitive yoga upon arriving at Menninger?*

Kayla: *When I got there, I couldn't stand to sit still. They gave me the calendar, which I was thrilled to get, and I looked over everything and noticed trauma-sensitive yoga, which really piqued my curiosity. I mentioned it to my social worker, and she said, "Why don't you talk to your psychiatrist about it?" So I asked to be put in within the first week of being there.*

Jessica: *What do you think piqued your interest about it?*

Kayla: *Well, I love yoga and I also believed in the benefits of it. And I knew that I was a trauma patient, and I had never heard of it, so I was curious to see more about it.*

Jessica: *And you've done a lot of yoga, Pilates, other body-focused exercises in your life? What's been your experience with that?*

Kayla: *I have worked with a personal trainer three times a week doing Pilates on and off, with my pregnancies being difficult, for eight years. It's just always been a healing practice for me. I liked the way I felt, I liked the way I looked after. Yoga was something I had done years ago and had put away because I felt it was doing harm to my arms and shoulders. When this came up when I was there [at Menninger], I wanted to take advantage of everything that was offered.*

Jessica: *What were your initial reactions to the class?*

Kayla: *When I first got in the class, Dallas said, "This yoga has been shown to decrease the effects of trauma by 33 percent," and I thought, wow. If that's true, that's incredible. Then he got into the poses, and at first he was saying, "It's your body; you can do what you want." I thought, "I get it. I get the game. We're supposed to feel empowered. I get it." I went through it anyway, and it was still kind of enjoyable and peaceful, and I thought, "If these benefits are true, I'm sticking with it."*

At one point, my social worker was trying to make my family therapy call during that time, and we had to explain that you have to have a certain number of sessions to be really effective. We reworked part of my schedule to allow me to stay in there.

Jessica: *I remember after you had been to several sessions, you came into individual therapy and said you had felt a shift from "oh, we're supposed to feel empowered" to "okay, I will be empowered," and you did a different pose from what was suggested. Do you remember that?*

Kayla: *Oh my gosh, it's like emblazoned on my brain. Somehow Dallas saying that ["you can do what you want to with your body"] over and over sort of wormed its way into my subconscious. I didn't know that I wasn't already empowered. I didn't realize that it was okay for me to do something slightly different. And one day, he did a pose, and I thought, "I'm not doing that. I'm doing something else." Then I was thinking, "Oh my gosh, I'm doing another pose. I'm not doing everything everyone else is doing." It gave me a sense of pride. It started helping me find my words again. Find my voice. Find my soul.*

Jessica: *It seemed that for you it was figuring out the difference between empowerment and control, because control was so important for you and made you feel like you had power. This sense of doing everything like other people and doing everything right was different from "no, I'm going to do what my body wants and what I want," and that was very different for you.*

Kayla: *Very different, yeah.*

Jessica: *We talked in therapy about this mask of confidence that you put on. It made you feel good to have it on; you had it all together, you knew how to talk to people, and you knew what to say. I wonder what it was like to bring that into trauma-sensitive yoga and being told do what's under that mask; do what's right.*

Kayla: *Like I said, I met that with some cynicism. It was one of the moments where I thought, "I'm smart, I know what I'm doing, I get it," but I thought I would stick with it. I like yoga. It was calming, it was a quiet place, and I thought, "if nothing else, this is relaxing for me." Really and truly, that fourth or fifth session is when I had that light-bulb moment.*

Jessica: *Do you feel that carried through the rest of your sessions, or did you have to keep coming back to it and reminding yourself?*

Kayla: *I think it carried through the sessions, and it carried throughout my day at Menninger. There would also be a day here or there where I didn't want to make my own decisions, and it was nice to have someone just tell me to get in tree pose, and that was peaceful, too. It was sort of a journey and not necessarily linear.*

Jessica: *When reading about trauma-sensitive yoga, the idea of doing what your body is telling you it wants made me think of you. I think you've spent a lot of time either ignoring what your body is telling you to give in to someone else or giving in too much to what your body is asking for, like staying in bed all day. How was finding that balance?*

Kayla: *It was painful, because all of a sudden, my past unfolded before me of how many things I had put myself through and done in the name of trying to be perfect and not upset anybody. At times, I had confidence, and it wasn't just a mask. I felt confident. And at other times, I look back and just want to shake myself. When I dated guys in my teenage years, I was fairly promiscuous. It wasn't because I wanted to have sex with these guys. I honestly believed that they loved me and that I didn't want to upset them. It's so sad for me to say that out loud now—that I actually allowed that to happen to me. I wore too-small shoes for a year, because I felt my feet looked better at that size. That's how severe or significant it was, and I didn't even realize it.*

Jessica: *That's a really powerful parallel for trauma-sensitive yoga, because you went from not being worth anything if you don't do everything right to being worth something even if you do nothing right.*

Kayla: *And that's something I was never taught.*

Jessica: *Do you feel like it impacted your ability to engage in individual therapy with me?*

Kayla: *I don't know that I would say the two were necessarily related.*

Jessica: *Or vice versa?*

Kayla: *I think the first week I met with you, one of the things you asked me was what I was most proud of. You strategically did that as I was about to leave the session, thinking, "Well, that was easy," and you said, "Just one more question—what's your biggest accomplishment?" And I stared at you with a blank stare, speechless, and I am never speechless. And that really bothered me, and you said, "Yeah, that's something we need to work on." I made it my goal, my dharma, that I needed to do whatever I needed to do to feel me again.*

Jessica: *What was your experience with the other people in the trauma-sensitive yoga class?*

Kayla: *Some of it was camaraderie. There were a few from the young adult unit, and I felt very motherly toward them, because I'm kind of a natural mom. There was one person that was very distracting to me, and I even described her as the thorn in my trauma yoga side. Through training and my therapy, I was able at some point to start to have compassion for her. At first I would think, "Please don't come back; you're stressing me out," and as time went on I just accepted that she was going to be there. She may have needed it more than I did. I came to a place of acceptance where I was just glad she had a place to go.*

Jessica: *That's huge, because chaos is hard for you, and that was a chaotic and uncontrollable thing. To come to a place of peace with it, and that was something we talked about a lot, that peace was very important to you, and it felt like unless your environment was peaceful, you couldn't find peace. But in this case, you found it in an unpeaceful environment.*

Kayla: *Yes, and we were having all these classes on mindfulness and mentalizing [according to psychologist Jon G. Allen, mentalizing is the "quality of explicitly and implicitly recognizing the mental states of others and oneself"[3]], and it was being able to look at someone with different eyes. It helped me tune her out and focus on my mat and what I was getting from it.*

Dallas: *It sounds like you were able to make a really conscious decision about "I want to do this differently."*

Kayla: *Yes. There was an older person also in treatment who had such a positive attitude, and they went to everything, and they got good things from everything. They said, "You get what you put into it." I thought about it, and I've just entered so many things in my life with cynicism. Like I knew the outcome already, or it was just going to be dumb like five other things I had done. Somewhere in my treatment early on, I thought, "I am going to take advantage of everything that is offered and know that I am going to glean something good from it." Whether the teacher's crummy or classmates irritate me or group therapy makes me want to run*

out of the room screaming, there is something to learn from everything,
and I made it my mission to do that.

Dallas: *When you made the change with the trauma-sensitive yoga, I wonder*
if you sort of saw yourself with new eyes, not unlike you saw the other
[difficult] member of the class.

Kayla: *It was if a black veil had been lifted off of me. I could feel a white rose*
starting to open up again and to start over this rebirth of being able to see
myself as a kind person. Being able to see myself as a good mother. Being
able to see myself as someone who encourages others. I had not had those
feelings of confidence in my true being or my soul maybe ever. That analogy
of the white rose is very specific to me; earlier I was meditating, and I was
thinking about how I just feel like a new person. In my life now, as it was
at Menninger from week to week, I'm improving in ways I didn't know were
possible. I feel like I'm becoming anew, and I feel like I'm presenting myself
to the people who matter as a person who is without bondage and without
too much baggage. Or some baggage, but has worked their way through it.

Dallas: *I'm in awe of that. What did you share about your experience with*
trauma-sensitive yoga while you were participating?

Kayla: *I mostly talked with my husband about it; he usually got the day-by-*
day replay. I told him I was doing this yoga, and I was glad, but so far I
couldn't really see how it was different from yoga. I quoted that statistic
at him, and I said, "If that's true, I absolutely need to take advantage
of this." I also remember telling him when that day happened, when I
shifted mindsets, and I said, "I get it. I get it now, and I'm so glad I
decided to stay."

Dallas: *Taking effective action is learning something from your body, then*
using that information to take some kind of action based on that knowl-
edge in concrete ways. For example, you might discover that if you're in a
twist, you can sort of figure out, "How much do I want to twist? What does
that feel like? Do I want to change that in some way, more of that, less of
that, differently?" Then, following through on that is taking that process
of effective action. I'm wondering about your experience with that.

Kayla: *So part of my case with trauma is that it presented with somatic pain. I went for a year hurting all over, being checked out by every doctor, and not finding an answer. That's when we started to think something might be going on in my brain, and that's when we started therapy and medication. So I came into Menninger with somatic pain, and it felt like a mountain I couldn't climb. I was trying to learn how to identify the pain, figure out what was causing it, and work my way through it using the tools that I had. When I came into yoga, I think that manifested in a couple of different ways, mentally and physically.*

Physically, the more I did TSY, the more I was able to feel what my body wanted to feel, or what I thought would feel good, or what I thought it needed more of. Like I thought it would feel good if I stretched this leg a little longer or sat in this particular position, and it helped me take control over my body and the senses I was allowing my body to feel. Once I started identifying what was happening, that was a huge component in learning how to get more in touch with my body. Instead of thinking, "I feel horrible pain, and I feel anxious, but I don't know why," now I could say, "I feel pain, and I feel it right here, and it's because I feel anxious because of this, this, and this." And it isn't a catastrophe, and I can deep-breathe and work my way through it. Mentally, the person I mentioned in the class was challenging, and I thought, "I can't change them, and I can't make it go away, but I can block them out."

Jessica: *Taking action without knowing if it's effective was something that could be really powerful for you. To trust that you might do something that won't work, and that's okay, and then you try something else.*

Kayla: *It makes you more adaptable.*

Dallas: *The ability to be adaptable, to be flexible, is so important. Both chronic pain and trauma leave us kind of rigid, so with yoga you end up being adaptable at different levels.*

Kayla: *Well, I can't take too much credit for that. One thing that is just a gift and one of my top five strengths is adaptability. I think this is a really good way and a saving grace way to be able to use it. I'm thankful I have a natural inclination towards that. It also helped me be able to say and do what I needed again. That was huge for me, because I would let people stress me out to where I would give in in a negotiation, or I would be put in an awkward position, because I wouldn't say, "You know, I don't want to talk about this." I used to have the ability to do that, but I lost touch with that over the past seven or eight years. So it helped me get my grip back.*

Dallas: *That's amazing.*

Kayla: *I know—it's amazing what it did for me.*

Dallas: *And you let it expand through all areas of your life.*

Kayla: *Yes.*

Dallas: *What was hard about the classes or anything about the classes or the process for you?*

Kayla: *You know, I don't know that there was too much about it that was hard. I did feel a little claustrophobic in that space. I wanted to be able to spread out a little more. Other than that, I was happy in there. I felt that was where I needed to be.*

Jessica: *One thing I was wondering about was what you brought to the class. It's never a one-directional thing; every person in that class got something different. I'm wondering what you brought to the class that helped it to be so impactful to you. You talked about adaptability. What else do you think you contributed to make that such an important therapy for you?*

Kayla: *I found this across the board at Menninger, what a strong mother instinct I have. I say that because half the reason I ended up there is because I felt like a bad mom. What I found was I'm a good natural mother; what I've got is a difficult situation, and a bunch of kids, and they're really little, and that's hard on anybody. Not every mother falls into the June Cleaver box, not every mother is the craft mom or the go and do the jump house mom. It's cool if I'm the Witch of Eastwick mom, and I know my kids and I know the best way to love and validate them.*

Jessica: *And you're the best mom for them.*

Kayla: *Yeah.*

Dallas: *Again, that's really being in tune with who you are and trusting that "I know this, I'll be okay, I can do this whatever this is."*

Kayla: *And that's been a journey. It didn't happen overnight, and I still consistently work on it. At one point I was thinking about how independent we all are, and thought maybe it's such a huge blessing. The fact that I'm independent and do my own thing and love on them, but I'm off creating my own things as well, might be the best combination I can be for them.*

Dallas: *Absolutely. It gives them space and models at the same time.*

Kayla: *Absolutely.*

Dallas: *Well, this has been such a learning opportunity for me, and I appreciate your willingness to take this on and be so candid.*

Kayla: *I was thrilled to participate. Thank you.*

The authors learned so much from this conversation and this chapter. Kayla's experience with TCTSY filtered throughout her experience at Menninger as a whole. She worked through issues from her life in TCTSY and issues from TCTSY in the rest of her treatment. Kayla's experience with taking effective action—moving her body in a way that felt good and right to her—helped her reclaim ownership in a way that she hadn't known she was missing. This conversation highlights the exquisite complexity of the human experience; there were millions of interactions and moments that led to a team consisting of Kayla, Dallas, Sonia, and Jessica. The multidirectional impact of each person's decision can be traced through explorations like this chapter, and it helps us to be curious about our own mind and that of those around us.

As stated earlier, it is rare for facilitators to receive such nuanced feedback about a patient's growth through any group or therapy, and it is rare for patients to hear about their providers' minds when engaged in treatment; simply put, we just don't know much of what's happening in each other's minds. For both providers of and participants in TCTSY, the skill of taking effective action is highly valuable when sitting with considerable discomfort regarding not-knowing: Given what I know, what can I do that serves my values the most? The values we serve by offering this chapter are growth, genuineness, and contribution; even though we don't know how it will be received or whether there was a more powerful, interesting, or exciting way to write it, we know that we've served our values by sharing it.

> I'm currently training to be a registered yoga teacher. This incredibly difficult and life-altering time in my life allowed me to find my dharma, or purpose. I plan to pursue a position where I can share the gift of yoga with other people who are struggling with addiction or mental health troubles.
>
> I was given the opportunity to save my own life. I feel called to lead others to healing and to help them remember who THEY are and that THEIR lives are absolutely worth saving. —Kayla

Relearning and Rewriting

Young Adults Claim Their Healing

Angelica Emery-Fertitta

FOR YOUNG PEOPLE WHO HAVE experienced developmental trauma, choice-making based on their own needs can be a foreign and often unavailable concept. Young adults and children are frequently given very little room for their voices to be heard. This is especially true in environments such as schools, group care settings, foster care, and inpatient psychiatric treatment centers. The experience of being a minor can lead to compounding experiences of coercion, ineffectiveness, and manipulation, particularly for young people with complex intersections of identity that lead to ongoing systemic oppression.

These coercive experiences occur in both big and small ways. Although these experiences can lead to ongoing challenges in mental, physical, and behavioral health, they are often overlooked and accepted as the norm. When an individual is attended to and surrounded by systems that overlook young people's voice and choice, this experience can become internalized. The message for the young person can be: "It doesn't matter what I feel or what I want because things will happen differently anyway—I am not in control of my body or my experience, and there is nothing I can do to change that." While this internalized experience is likely to lead to long-term consequences in terms of well-being and outcomes, opportunities for developing self-efficacy are not generally prioritized in the care and therapeutic treatment of youths. In Trauma Center Trauma-Sensitive

Yoga (TCTSY), this need is addressed by practicing noticing, making sense of, and then responding to sensations in one's own body—that is, taking effective action.

For the entirety of my career, I have served young people in settings like those mentioned earlier. I have witnessed young people's experiences of being confined, ignored, and coerced into doing activities, or pushed into ways of being. Some of these actions we take for granted, such as the moments when we ask a child to sit still or be quiet while their body and mind are requesting movement. Other incidents are larger and systemic in nature. Young people have little say when it comes to courses of action related to their removal from parents or guardians and subsequent placement. I have also witnessed young people with profound insight into the mental health care and approach that would serve them best in moments of crisis. Yet they are often told that the provider knows better or that their advocacy is appreciated but the adults are looking at moving in a different direction.

The issue is complex because for young people there are certainly times when adults have the experience and vantage point of being able to see beyond the particular moment the youth may be focused on. But the youth's experience of being ineffective at getting their needs met, or feeling helpless and out of control, is sustained. For example, a young adult, age sixteen, sits in a provider meeting and advocates for why residential care is no longer useful in her treatment. She makes an argument for the support that she believes would better serve her in the community and why it is more likely to lead to her ongoing success. The adults in the room listen. Some are even impressed. But, ultimately, the decision is made behind closed doors that her caregiver is not able to provide the support she needs at this time because of the caregiver's own mental health concerns. The providers likely have her best interests in mind; and there are dynamics at play that may be challenging for the young person to hear or integrate. Still, when this is communicated to her, she is likely to walk away with a feeling that no matter how self-aware, mature, or clear she is about what is best for her, she will not be heard.

These moments always remind me of Judith Herman's quote, "No intervention that takes power away from the survivor can possibly foster her recovery, no matter how much it appears to be in her immediate best interest."[1] This way of understanding trauma and interventions for those who have experienced trauma leads to the question of how we begin to foster experiences of effective action. In other words, when a young person notices a sensation or a need, could they be given space to respond to it in a way that matches the need and resolves the need? This can happen in small- or large-scale moments. In the previous example, could the young person's perspective be validated? Could she be brought into the solution? In this particular instance, perhaps going home to the identified caregiver isn't an option; but could we team with this young person to uncover a solution that meets the concerns she has brought forward? In my experience, I have found embodiment to be a useful opportunity for practicing this skill of responding to personal needs and developing a sense of efficacy and subsequent empowerment for a young person. In this sense, it might look like engaging in a yoga practice with a young person. They may notice pain in their leg when they move a certain way and decide to voice this. If they are then given the space to adjust the way they are moving to respond to that sensation in a way that feels useful to them, they have an opportunity to take effective action.

I have had the opportunity to offer TCTSY to young people in a variety of settings and formats. I have, for example, offered TCTSY to youths in brief individual sessions within a residential care setting north of Boston. This program serves youths age sixteen to twenty-two and prepares them for independent living. In a setting like this, the experiences of trauma, as well as family separation and major mental illness, are ubiquitous. These settings also enforce immense structure and often rely on behavioral interventions as well as restraints and/or police response to manage larger safety incidents. Many activities are mandated to maintain privilege status, meaning that there is little opportunity for choice and a sense of control. Although it varies from setting to setting, privileges are earned and lost. These privileges include being able to go out into the community, participate in preferred activities, and have independent time outside of the residence. Privileges are earned by attending and fully participating in therapeutic groups, by going to bed on time, by completing hygiene, and by generally following the community guidelines and expectations. For example, a young person who struggles to take showers on a daily basis or brush their teeth twice a day might be put on "holding," which could prohibit them from taking the afternoon trip to the mall. Or if a youth identifies that the therapeutic boxing group is overwhelming to her and she does not participate, she may again be held from participating in preferred activities later that day or the next. In a setting like this, yoga based on invitational language and choice-making can initially be quite confusing, for staff and young people alike.

In order to introduce myself and this unique approach, I began by holding a house meeting where we discussed past experiences with yoga (many young people have been exposed to brief yoga interventions at higher levels of care, such as Community-Based Acute Treatment programs). Youths identified that they weren't the right "type" of person to do yoga, that they didn't like being told to move slowly and be quiet, or that they had found yoga made them anxious. I made space for these experiences, acknowledged the validity of them, and then offered some background on how this approach to yoga *might* look or feel different.

My first day back at the program after the group meeting, a few youths self-selected to come by. They began with short sessions where they chose yoga cards. They also chose the way they would interact with these forms. Some of the options I offered included practicing on the mat or in a chair, linking movements or keeping them separate, music or no music, and style of music. This last choice led to a lot of excitement, especially for young people who did not feel personally or culturally connected to commonly used relaxation music. Eventually more youths became interested in interacting with TCTSY, especially when they heard from their peers that they got to make choices about almost every aspect of the practice. A young woman of Guatemalan heritage, for example, chose music that was sung in Spanish and traditional to her culture. While listening to this music, she selected specific forms and got excited about trying more physically engaging forms. She ended up sharing this experience with her friends, which led others to be more interested in exploring this opportunity as well. This was the first time I had offered an option beyond music or no music. I was struck by the importance and the beauty of moving beyond this A/B choice to better incorporate young people's cultural experiences, preferences, and knowledge of what works for them. I felt immense appreciation and humility for how adjusting one small aspect of a practice can lead to an entirely different experience for the participant. By sharing power in this way, the young woman was able to shape the practice into something she wanted and was able to engage with.

I had the chance to work with many young people in this setting, but one young man in particular stands out. He sat in the back during the initial meeting with his hood on and his eyes closed. He had his chair tilted precariously on the back two legs, propped against the wall. He chose not to attend the first few weeks but always seemed to be checking out the yoga room by just being around. He would pop his head in now and then or just wander by. I regularly observed him talking with staff or his peers using expletives. He would puff out his chest and engage in physically aggressive "play." He walked with a heaviness to his gait, shifting slightly side to side as he moved forward in space. In my observations of the group dynamics, he presented as someone who others both feared and admired, offering him respect and following his lead.

I eventually learned that this young man had an extensive trauma history, had been involved with gangs, and was often getting into physical altercations. He did not engage in therapy and was not generally open to discussing his feelings or needs in the therapeutic milieu.

After about a month, he asked to try some yoga. He began by choosing several cards and then requesting five minutes of guided movements (based on the yoga cards) that were linked to one another as a cohesive practice. The length of time slowly increased, and after a few weeks he was requesting twenty- to thirty-minute individual sessions. His voice would be loud and his chest and chin raised as we walked toward the dining room that served as a yoga space. When we entered the room and closed the door, his shoulders would drop, as would the volume of his voice. He would begin by explaining how he had been feeling and what he believed he needed in his yoga session on that particular day. He requested long periods of resting at the end of the practice, as well as an opportunity to sit in stillness.

One day as we were closing the practice he looked up and said, "I just feel so peaceful when I am here . . . and I know . . . that if I want to be happy I need to find this peace more often. I need to share it too." His words were slow, thoughtful, and quiet, almost as if to himself. To me, this demonstrated the ultimate form of effective action, knowing what he wanted and needed in order to attain the life experience he desired. Beyond that, he was linking the feeling and knowledge to what he wanted to bring to the world around him. Once he had found his own body and the ability to befriend his body, he was able to connect with others around him in a new way.

After this moment, he began coming around with me asking his peers if they were interested in trying some yoga. Sometimes the staff would jump in saying things like, "Yeah! You guys need to do this and you need to participate fully. It's good for you." He would quickly reply, "Well it's actually your choice . . . It's more individual; it's different for each person."

I was blown away by the remarkable difference I was seeing from the young man I first met, and the way that he was fully experiencing his ability to understand his body and make choices based on his own experiences. When it came time for him to move toward independent living, he requested drawings of the series of forms we often explored. He took them with him, stating that this way, he could find peace wherever he ended up.

Another format for this practice was offering weekly group yoga sessions at a nonprofit organization located in Boston. This organization, which has a wide range of programming, serves low-income women and youths from the Boston area who have lost family members to community violence. Youths who were deemed "at-risk" for involvement in community violence or who had lost siblings to violence were invited to join after-school and summer programming where trauma-sensitive yoga sessions were integrated.

Initially the youths (ages fifteen to eighteen) were skeptical, raising their eyebrows and explaining that yoga was not for them. Their exposure to yoga was Instagram influencers who looked and lived nothing like they did. The majority of the folks they had seen were white, thin, and wealthy—living in what appeared to be luxurious conditions. Their reality didn't match this. Most of the youths in this group identified as Black or Latinx, represented a wide range of body types, and came from families who experienced financial instability. As a white woman with an athletic build, my presence in some ways enhanced this skepticism and led to an even greater differentiation in power from "student" to "teacher" based on my privileged identities. It was important for me to verbally acknowledge this dynamic, highlighting that although we may have different identities and yoga is often presented in this one way in the US, this practice can be available to any body. I took this opportunity to explore the roots of yoga practice and how it was not originally created for or by wealthy white women. Through conversation, relationship building, and an emphasis on demonstrating my desire to share power, I worked to actively engage in breaking down the perception and dynamic of Western yoga norms that yoga is for thin, white, wealthy, and temporarily able-bodied people. My goal in this process was not to convince them that this perception or dynamic was untrue; rather, I attempted to acknowledge the ways that these norms are problematic and then explore where and how the youths might find a space to engage with this practice in a way that worked for them. In this instance, it was important that I be transparent while working collaboratively to develop community.

The sessions began with a check-in where youths had the opportunity to introduce themselves, their current energy level, and how their week had been. We began with some seated forms and eventually made our way to standing, at which point youths were invited to utilize yoga cards to participate in shaping the session. These sessions were initially filled with laughter, giggling, and side conversations. By acknowledging that this new way of moving and being together can be funny, I was able to welcome this into the space. I also used the laughter and conversation as a tool to increase engagement and demonstrate my desire to share power with the youths by avoiding any assertion of authority in these moments. After several meetings, youths began to take the sessions a bit more seriously and engage in them in a new way. This happened naturally and by demonstrating shared power, rather than by forced participation or coercion. In some settings, you might see adults encouraging youths to engage in the practice in a certain way. This can range from something like "this will help your anxiety" to "if you engage with this, we can go out and get ice cream later" or "you have to be quiet and listen to what the adult tells you to do." In contrast, participants here were welcomed to engage in a way that worked for them each session. Sometimes this meant finding stillness. Other times this meant going to a different part of the room and drawing, while some days it meant moving through forms. The possibility of noticing sensation in their bodies at the present moment, or interoception, was offered along with some of these forms and movements.

At the end of each session, I offered space for youths to provide input and feedback, reminding them that the goal was for the sessions to feel useful to them. In order to make this more accessible to all styles, I offered space for verbal as well as anonymous written feedback. Presenting these options is important, because although I work to create a space of shared power, an innate power dynamic exists in any experience with a facilitator, especially when the facilitator is an adult and the participants are young people. There can be fear associated with giving feedback (even when it is invited), sometimes based on past experiences. Feedback can be manipulated, distorted, or taken out of context and ultimately utilized as a means of causing or justifying harm to the person who offered it. Many of these young people have also had experiences where they lacked control, so it was a priority to develop opportunities for feedback as a form of co-creation. By presenting options for co-creating this space, we were able to support the rebuilding of these young people's sense of empowerment of their own bodies and, eventually, in their lives. Another important piece of sharing power and demonstrating consistency was to seek their input on any shifts or changes to "business as usual," actively incorporating suggestions as they were offered.

Eventually, young people became so invested that they requested to facilitate the opening or closing of the session. (This portion of the session was always consistent.) They would even facilitate using similar language, offering invitations and the opportunity to make choices. This was a powerful moment as a facilitator. It provided me with direct feedback that my work to share power and my conscientious use of language had been received by the participants. It demonstrated to me that they were in a place of embodied empowerment. The opportunity to witness this growth and this desire to replicate the experience for one another was awe inspiring. I found a sense of quiet and joy as I listened to the young people take charge of their practice and their space.

The staff were also excited to share with me that youths were discussing the benefits of the sessions in between meetings. The youths explained that the practice felt helpful, as it provided them with some time to relax their bodies and get focused; and they were excited to have the opportunity to practice some of their favorite parts of the practice between sessions when they felt it would be useful to them. It is important to note again that they did this of their own volition. Instead of instructing youths on what shapes to make, and when and how to make them, I presented opportunities to make choices and connections. Sometimes youths are told what will make them calm or what will make them feel better. In these sessions, I noticed that, given the tools as well as the opportunity to have ownership over their bodies and engage in interoception, they made these choices for themselves.

As the sessions continued, the variety of ways that youths chose to engage with the practice grew. Sometimes this was with stillness, subtle movements, and quiet. Other days, youths chose to be more active, engaging their muscles and playing choice-based yoga games. One example of these games included using a large dice and a chart with different yoga forms. The youths would take turns rolling the dice. The number the dice landed on corresponded to two possible yoga forms on the chart. Youths had the opportunity to select one of these forms or to create their own. There was then the possibility for the youths either to guide the group through the form or request my assistance with that component. Games like this created an opportunity for sessions to be more interactive and fast paced for days where slower, meditative movement was not as accessible. A game like this allows for making choices, exploring forms, and noticing sensations in a way that engages play and might feel more natural to young people.

The emphasis on choice-making and interoceptive awareness paved the way for varied experiences from session to session. The more we practiced together, the more youths' voices grew, evidence of their increasing sense of empowerment and self-efficacy. They came together and advocated for changes in the structure and content of the sessions. At this point in time, sessions were being offered on Friday afternoons prior to some vocational work. Youths advocated that they would prefer the sessions close out their day and week as a way to "start the weekend more connected to their minds and bodies." They explained that they had been talking about how hard it was to transition from yoga to work at the end of a long week. They concluded that it would be more useful to meet after their vocational time.

Based on this feedback, I worked with the program to accommodate this request. When we made the shift, youths reported increased satisfaction and benefit. According to them, this benefit included feeling empowered to make safer choices throughout the weekend because they felt more "grounded." This was particularly significant because these suggestions (and outcomes) were theirs and theirs alone. This sense of ownership over the practice appeared to be very powerful for them.

Throughout these sessions, participants were provided the space and time to begin to notice sensations in their body in the moment (e.g, saying "oh, I feel this stretch in my leg!" or "this side feels different than the other"). The sessions offered an opportunity to move and focus on their bodies. They also offered space to explore finding quiet in a supportive environment, one characterized by camaraderie, exploration, and curiosity. While these youths came with different life stories, they made a choice to show up and engage with one another in a shared and novel experience that they otherwise might not have felt was accessible to them. This experience was uniquely theirs, thereby creating space to engage with what may have previously felt foreign.

As participants were exploring the opportunity to take effective action related to the sensations and needs of their own bodies ("this hurts my back, so I am going to do this version instead"), they were beginning to regain empowerment and an embodied sense of self. Many of these youths had previous experiences where they were not able to take action to resolve discomfort, whether in their bodies, minds, or interpersonally. For example, young people who experienced physical abuse at the hands of adults may not have been able to protect themselves from harm in the moment. Or a young person who witnessed the mistreatment of their caregiver may not have had the chance, the physical ability, or the tools to protect them. This can lead to feeling disjointed, ineffective, fearful, or agitated. Having the opportunity to restore a sense of control can pave the way to feeling physically, psychologically, and emotionally integrated.

A core component of traumatic experiences, particularly familial and/or developmental trauma, is loose interpersonal boundaries or disrespected boundaries. These experiences can enforce a sense that in order to be in relationship or community with others you must adapt, blend in, and be the same, losing your sense of individuality. These young people began to emphasize choice-making and their uniqueness to one another by highlighting the fact that "this [a forward fold] makes me feel calm, but my friend said that it makes her anxious. So she does this [bows her head] instead." The process allowed them to have and highlight different experiences, while remaining in relationship and in community. One way of being was not right and the other was not wrong. The two (or three or more) different ways could coexist and even be celebrated.

The sense of empowerment and embodiment led to change outside the yoga sessions as well. Although this was not something we discussed, the young people organically took the experience of effective action outside of the four walls of their after-school program. This included engaging in advocacy efforts in their community to reduce the factors that lead to violence, not only identifying what was wrong in their eyes but proposing and advocating for ways to make things better. Their engagement in the community demonstrated effective action on a large scale: noticing an issue, suggesting a resolution, and taking action to achieve the desired outcome.

The opportunity to practice moving, practice noticing sensations, and practice making choices based on these sensations, eventually achieving a preferred outcome, can lead to the development or redevelopment of important skills lost through the experience of interpersonal or institutional trauma. By stepping out of the way of young people, by offering choices and opportunities for embodiment, I was able to support, but not prescribe, the development of effective action. Effective action is a skill and a tool for navigating the nuances and complexities of life. This skill can be taken out of the yoga room and into the world. Young people can learn to notice something, whether it is a sensation, a need, a want, or a problem, and then decide how they want to move forward to make a change that leads to a more desirable outcome. With this knowledge and ability, a young person may experience a sense of empowerment and a sense of being effective as they engage in the world around them. The ability to take skilled, knowledgeable, and successful action—with a sense of empowerment—can support young people as they transition to adulthood and engage in their own process of healing and growth.

Taking Assertive Action

Group Therapy off the Mat

Christine Cork

THIS IS THE STORY OF the first group I facilitated that incorporated Trauma Center Trauma-Sensitive Yoga (TCTSY). I work in a group psychiatric practice that in addition to medication management offers psychological testing and psychotherapy. We are social workers, marriage and family therapists, mental health counselors, psychologists, and psychiatrists all working together. There are two main hospital systems in town, but we are independent and make our own practice decisions as we belong to neither medical system. We can see a variety of clients based on our interests and have the autonomy to see clients based on need, as we are able. In this clinical setting, I operate primarily as a therapist to adolescents and adults. I wanted to offer a group that was useful to clients in a different way than groups I have facilitated in the past. Trained in offering psychoeducational groups, where I talk, and process groups, where everybody talks, I wanted to offer TCTSY, which does not rely on talking.

Trauma-specific talk therapy offers some relief from trauma response symptoms, but it does not always give clients as much freedom as they would like. There are specific trauma therapies that address symptoms such as flashbacks and nightmares with exposure and changing cognitions that emerge out of the traumatic incident, but TCTSY offers the body a chance to process, to embody the feelings and sensations, and possibly to let them go. TCTSY offers the possibility of interoception, an awareness of internal body sensations. I was intrigued with the possibility that trauma survivors could own their bodies again after being made to feel powerless in them. This is the freedom of experience that I believe talk therapy does not always get to, and I have known many brave and hardworking people over the years who have come so far to be functional and useful in their lives to others but still have very little to do with their bodies. I think of one client in particular who showers as quickly as she can, trying to be unaware of what she is doing when she is cleaning her body. Trauma sometimes leads to ignoring or distancing from the body so you do not have to be aware of it. The body, in this case, was the thing that allowed my client to be hurt, and being vulnerable without clothes even with a locked door was terrifying. Showering every other day is a triumph over avoidance and quickly exhausts her. To be completely transparent, I wanted to see for myself if this adjunctive treatment for complex trauma was as useful as the research indicated it could be. I wanted to see if clients could reconnect with their bodies in adaptive ways.

The science of my discipline is very important to me. I try to offer things that are research based because I do not want to mislead people. I know that anecdotal evidence is not sufficient to demonstrate that something will be useful to people in general, and I never want to be lumped with those who convince others they are improving through charm and sheer force of will. These victories would be hollow to me as they are not true victories, just manipulation of people who are desperate for answers and relief. I have heard stories from clients who end up feeling betrayed, abandoned, and perpetually damaged after a religious leader, health-care provider, or homeopathic guide offered a solution for all their troubles and they failed to get better. They were compliant but ended up feeling that the fault was theirs because the authority was so certain that they were right about someone else's experience. Yoga has been important to me in my life because it has improved my relationship and attention to my body. Intuitively it made sense to me that it might help my clients, but I did not offer it as intervention until I saw the scientific evidence. It was also important to me to see it in practice, so I could be as trustworthy as possible. In order to recommend a strategy in therapy, I need to know the research, be prepared and trained in the technique, and have some personal experience and supervision with the strategy. Then I can be genuine in offering the possibility to my clients and congruent in having the best interest of my client in mind.

Therefore, I planned. This trustworthy thing is not something I take lightly. I work very hard at it, and I wanted to have consistency for my participants. Trauma survivors have enough experience with chaos. Inconsistent adults, rules changing between public and private, not knowing if you were going to get hurt, and having no expectation of safety. It was important to me that the group would feel as safe as possible. I like to be predictable, dependable, and well trained. Growing up with a parent who was unpredictable and frequently too overwhelmed with her own stuff to be available and competent with me has left its mark. I endeavor to be the solid one in the therapeutic relationship. Personally I like a bit of flexibility and spontaneity. I do things in my own time and in my own way on the weekends. During the week, I bring the flexibility but also make a point of being on time and ending on time with clients. It is a matter of respect and provides a consistent container for the experience. They know what to expect of me.

I needed to decide on time, day, and location and coordinate with my practice. Things can get busy and noisy in the hallways, and I wanted to find a space with limited interruption. If I was going to use an open office for the group, I needed to communicate with the others in the practice so the room would no longer be used as everyone's closet. I wanted the room to be quiet, private, and known so that we did not get any unexpected visitors during group. We needed enough space for the group so that participants would not feel crowded. They needed to have their own space. I decided to host the group on an evening when the practice was open but there were fewer providers in the building. This would cut down on noise and the possibilities of interruption. In addition it would support the office staff in maintaining work-life balance, as I was not asking them to remain after hours for just my group and me. I distributed handouts to each provider giving them a sense of what I was doing with the group and when I would be offering it. I also made handouts for possible participants so they had something to read when they got home for additional information.

For the providers, I highlighted what TCTSY was and what it was not. In the beginning I was approached by some who wanted to refer into my group for relaxation training or as an opportunity for physical activity. Both of those are helpful to clients, but TCTSY is hard work and, for many trauma survivors, not relaxing. It was very important to set appropriate expectations: TCTSY may be helpful, and a client would need to be prepared for it and connected with a therapist before beginning. I gave information about my training and included websites if they wanted to look at the research themselves. For the participants, I noted the time and place, and I highlighted that participants, including me, would stay on their mat. They would not have to worry about touch, and the practice was doable. I reminded them that they did not need special clothing or equipment and that they could contact me if they had questions or concerns. I invited participants who were clients of mine for the first group. My plan was to open the group after this first experience, but I wanted to have a relationship with these first participants. My thinking was that if I already knew them and they knew me, I would have more access to feedback during the process.

I kept the group small, and I wanted this experience to have a start and end so that I could gather data. My intent was to facilitate a ten-week pilot group (like the NIH study at the Trauma Center), and I invited those who I believed would be interested out of my own caseload. I was clear that for this group I was inviting participants who were female. This was also a safety consideration. Group met weekly for sixty minutes, and we spent the first half participating in movement together using the TCTSY framework. We then had a voluntary activity to participate in that highlighted coping skills. I asked participants to complete the Post-Traumatic Stress Disorder Checklist) before participating. It is a self-report checklist that asks about post-traumatic stress symptoms and their severity. It has military and civilian versions; my participants were civilians, so I used that version. I planned to offer the opportunity to complete one at the end of the experience as well. I let participants know that I would welcome feedback, as using TCTSY was a learning experience for me as well. In trauma work, it is essential to address the power dynamics in the relationship. Because helplessness and powerlessness are key components of the original trauma, I try to share power in the relationship, and welcoming feedback and participating myself are two opportunities. One of the reasons I was so drawn to TCTSY in the beginning was the acknowledgment of power dynamics in both yoga class and clinical settings. The model encourages the sharing of power and dismantling the embedded power structure of teacher-student and therapist-client. I wanted to offer collaboration and balance the relationship.

Two women accepted my invitation. Diana and Michelle were clients with depression and anxiety diagnoses. Both had survived sexual abuse perpetrated by a family member. Diana reported that she was anxious about work, made worse by a supervisor who was mercurial and critical. She expressed concern that doing something in the evening after work might overtax her already-overwhelmed self. She worried about her physical health and energy on a daily basis and focused on just getting to work and making it home because of her physical limitations. Michelle had escaped a physically abusive former partner. Michelle struggled with expressing her needs and wishes especially with authority figures. She acknowledged that she could be angry and direct, but she also worried that physicians would abandon her if she asked them for accommodations or options based on what was less traumatic for her. Michelle was also tired and frustrated at work. She acknowledged that she felt stuck. Both were married and worked full time. Both had done trauma work with therapists over the years and felt like they had made progress but continued to feel limited. They felt past trauma still claimed part of their lives and experiences.

These self-described limitations aside, they were very nice and competent people. They were kind and interested in others. These women would notice an outfit or haircut and offer support. They would also ask unbidden how I was doing, and it felt like they really wanted to know. Michelle was especially good at relating to and communicating with people in distress and helping them feel better. Diana was involved in caring for and rescuing animals. They were experts in their fields and knew their jobs well. They struggled with themselves, but they were compassionate with other people. They are amazing because of their struggles.

Both paused when asked about how it might feel to spend time with their bodies. They did not know. One shared that "I don't pay attention to my body." Another explained that the body was associated with memories of pain and shame, so she tried not to think about it or acknowledge it. Their courage was striking; they knew based on our conversations that TCTSY was a "body-based" intervention and they were willing to try it, even though it was unlike anything they had ever asked of themselves in therapy. I felt privileged, humbled, and responsible. I did not want to let them down, and thus began my struggle in staying present in the moment and being unattached to outcomes.

When I worry about my performance in a situation, I become less present. I know this from experience. The critic in my head can get in my way and pull me out of the experience. For this to work, I needed to be kind with myself and have no preconceived notions of what to expect. I want people to feel better. To have some relief or at least not get worse because of something that I did. Personally I have expectations that I am helpful to my clients. This is the reason I get up in the morning and go to work. The problem with personal expectations is that they are about me, my ego, and they can feel like pressure to others. Clients could feel like they have to get better in order for me to feel good about myself or be "good patients" if I leave my ego unchecked. My struggle is to be open to all possibilities without assumptions or judgments and stay curious. When this happens I can see, stay present, and offer what is truly helpful, not what makes me feel like I am helpful.

Our first evening, I went out into the lobby of the group practice that I work for, and we all headed back to an empty interior office lacking furniture. We had mats, a space, and participants. It was go-time, and the focus the first night was on me, or so I felt. It was very much like being observed when I was a terrified therapist-in-training and had multiple tracks running in my mind during session. I was anxious and did my best to offer a series of doable yoga forms, being very aware of my language. I wanted to offer an invitation or suggestions for movements, not commands. This is very different from a traditional yoga class and a different way of speaking when facilitating a group or even in an individual session. *If you like, perhaps,* and *maybe* introduce all sentences. Every movement introduced is a choice highlighted by the language that is used. It was awkward for me in the beginning because I was moving, monitoring my language, and trying to stay present. The critic got going in my head and started pointing out everything I was doing wrong. My ability to engage with my clients through shared authentic experience might have been sporadic. I noticed myself trying to be aware of my body in the moment, while also being very critical of my performance as a facilitator. I was not being kind to myself and fractured my experience in the process.

Both women were also apprehensive. I heard a nervous laugh or two and sometimes an *oomph* when moving into a shape that was less familiar to them. I had reviewed what to expect individually, but the experience is something else. Sometimes the movements are new experiences, and you have no idea how they work for your body. Sometimes sensations emerge from a part of your body that you are not used to hearing from, and the facilitator is asking you to listen. Everyone was quiet and very polite. We did sticky notes with a few words describing where we were at the end of practice. They thanked me for offering the group. On the first evening, I definitely felt that they were being kind and encouraging to me in offering gratitude. I resolved to be present and to be kind to myself as we continued.

I needed to get out of my head and into my body. I swim and I practice yoga outside of TCTSY, so this is where I started. I was participating in group supervision at the time, and I shared my challenges. The very helpful suggestion of giving myself time between my talk therapy sessions of the day and the group was accepted. I went into the group room early and reclined on the mat, giving myself time to attend to my own body and my own present moment awareness.

The second TCTSY session felt different. It felt like we were finding our rhythm and were more of three people in a room rather than a facilitator and two participants. It was a welcome experience for me to focus on sensations inside my body (interoception) instead of my self-observant critical voice that continually offers feedback if I allow it. The women started a routine of greetings and finding their space in the room. For an activity, I offered paper and crayons to draw safe spaces, real or imagined, for ourselves. I participated in the activity too, as I was reluctant to go back to being just the observer after feeling a connection during TCTSY practice.

As a therapist I am trained to maintain professional boundaries, but there is strength in joining that I was able to feel. Diana and Michelle were the experts in the room when it came to their experience and their bodies. I was there with mine. We were working on something together, and I was attempting to share power by practicing with them and being aware of me. I was careful to limit self-disclosure, but it was important for me to share as well. I could share about the experience in the room during group. Taking my turn, I was careful to welcome participation while expecting nothing other than what the women would choose to say and share about their drawings. I could voluntarily share my thoughts about the process and my drawing as well.

Our subsequent sessions continued to develop into this emergent rhythm, and then the most remarkable thing happened. My participants started asking questions of one another, talking to one another, and started setting goals for themselves outside of our room. I offered activities involving boundaries, mindfulness, self-compassion, grounding, and centering, but then the women would start addressing each other and including me when I wanted to join in the conversation. We had a conversation, and then we finished our time together.

The shift in power dynamics was palpable. I would work on staying present, inviting interoception, preparing a voluntary activity, and using invitatory language, and the women would take charge. I expected the opportunity for owning their bodies, but they owned the group. They asked about different forms and types of yoga. They had ideas for one another. They both found safety in outdoor images, and they suggested to one another that they could take break time outside of the building at work. They thought of things that they could make to help them focus and be mindful, like homemade glitter jars.

Then the stories of assertiveness outside of our room started emerging. Diana made a comment one night at the close of our practice. "I was worried about being tired after doing this at the end of day," she announced. "But I have been going home and doing stuff around the house. Weird." Michelle shared that she started putting personal objects that she could observe in her space at work to remind herself to be mindful and that she was safe. I got out of the way. It was clear that they were getting what they needed out of the practice. I did not need to show them the way. The emerging wisdom of my participants was delivering on what they needed. They had the insight into what would work for them.

Week by week, we continued to share movement and an activity, and the women would take action outside of the group. Michelle was assertive at work, requesting that she be accommodated for an active-shooter training at work. She did not want to attend the mandatory training because she had already had the experience of having a gun pointed at her head. She anticipated being triggered and asked for an alternate professional development activity. Her work accommodated without quibbling. Diana started attending family events, which she had avoided in the past. She asserted that she was no long afraid of running into specific family members because they know what they did and they should feel bad. She had been scared and ashamed when she thought about seeing them in person, but she realized that she had nothing to apologize for or feel bad about. Preparing options and emphasizing choices in individual sessions was also useful.

At our final session, Diana and Michelle completed the checklist again—they were surprised that their scores reflected considerable change. They had not noticed the diminishing of symptoms as much as the things they were doing in their lives. Diana was attending yoga, nature, and spirituality classes and was actively looking for things that interested her in the community. She made new friends and shared about herself. She started corresponding with the family members she felt comfortable with and traveled to graduations to witness the next generation of her family doing well. She was no longer tired at the end of the day and at the end of the week. She wanted more activity in her life. Michelle was thinking of things that could make her space at work more enjoyable and finding a way to make her hobby of making blankets into something that would benefit others.

I was amazed and humbled again. In some ways TCTSY feels so simple a practice. The physical movements were manageable for all in the room, and we did not challenge our strength, flexibility, or stamina. We did not have insight-driven conversations about the meaning of things. We just tried to experience them. The challenge is to stay present with yourself and with others to experience the body. As these women courageously chose to experience their bodies, they appeared to become more aware of the space that they needed in their lives and relationships.

My experience also changed. I got to witness two women grow in ways that none of us predicted. I started to call it "random acts of assertiveness" when asked what I had noticed about facilitating the group. It sounds a lot like taking effective action: using internal information like sensation, a feeling, or intuition through practicing interoception; to move differently in our bodies; or to make a change in our lives. It convinced the scientist and skeptic in me that TCTSY is a credible intervention. I knew this already, but I needed to prove it—feel it—for myself. It reminded the therapist that she does her best work when she gets out of the way, offers choices, and focuses on experiences. People do grow and change, but I do not have to be ego-invested in the outcomes. When clients take ownership of their bodies and processes for healing, the outcomes take care of themselves.

NOTES

Introduction

1 Babette Rothschild, *The Body Remembers* (New York: W.W. Norton, 2000).

2 Center for Disease Control and Prevention, "Adverse Childhood Experiences: Looking at How ACEs Affect Our Lives and Society," accessed April 10, 2020, https://vetoviolence.cdc.gov/apps/phl /images/ACE_Accessible.pdf.

3 Alison Rhodes, "Claiming Peaceful Embodiment through Yoga in the Aftermath of Trauma," *Complementary Therapies in Clinical Practice* 21 (2015): 251, http://www.traumacenter.org/products/pdf_files /Peaceful_Embodiment_Through_Yoga_R0002.pdf.

4 Rothschild, *The Body Remembers*, 45.

5 "Digging into Our Consciousness," *Los Angeles Times*, May 13, 2011, https://www.latimes.com/science/la-xpm-2011-may-13-la-sci -damasio-q-a-20110514-story.html.

6 Judith Herman, *Trauma and Recovery* (New York: Basic, 1992), 133.

7 Rhodes, "Claiming Peaceful Embodiment," 250.

Connecting in Safety

1 Eduardo Duran, *Healing the Soul Wound: Counseling with American Indians and Other Native Peoples* (New York: Teacher's College Press, 2006), 7.

Paralleled Agency

1 Center for Disease Control and Prevention, "What Is ME/CFS?," accessed February 29, 2020, https://www.cdc.gov/me-cfs/about/index.html.

2 Richard Tardif, "Research in CFS Opens a Door," updated November 19, 2019, http://richardtardif.com/research-into-cfs-opens-a-door/.

3 Jaime Seltzer and Julia Thomas, "ME Research Summary," accessed February 29, 2020, http://y9ukb3xprawlvtswp2e7ia6u-wpengine.netdna-ssl.com/wp-content/uploads/2019/06/19_MEA_Revised_2019_Research_Summary_190610.pdf.

4 Herman, *Trauma and Recovery*, 133.

5 Clare J. Fowler, "Visceral Sensory Neuroscience: Interoception," *Brain: A Journal of Neurology* 126, no. 6 (June 2003): 1505–1506.

6 *Merriam-Webster.com Dictionary*, s.v. "agency," accessed February 29, 2020, https://www.merriam-webster.com/dictionary/agency.

7 Anil K. Seth, Keisuke Suzuki, and Hugo D. Critchley, "An Interoceptive Predictive Coding Model of Conscious Presence," *Frontiers in Psychology* 2, no. 395 (January 10, 2012), https://doi.org/10.3389/fpsyg.2011.00395.

8 *Paperback Oxford English Dictionary*, s.v. "self" (Oxford, UK: Oxford University Press, 2012).

9 Noa Sadeh and Rachel Karniol, "The Sense of Self-Continuity as a Resource in Adaptive Coping with Job Loss," *Journal of Vocational Behavior* 80, no. 1 (2012): 93–99, https://doi.org/10.1016/j.jvb.2011.04.009.

10 Elisabeth Tova Bailey, *The Sound of a Wild Snail Eating* (Chapel Hill, NC: Algonquin Books, 2010), 131.

Authenticity in Vulnerability

1 National Capacity Building Project at the Center for Victims of Torture, "Working with Torture Survivors: Core Competencies," in *Healing the Hurt* (Minneapolis, MN: Center for Victims

of Torture, 2005), http://www.cvt.org/sites/default/files/u11/Healing_the_Hurt_Ch3.pdf.

2 National Capacity Building Project, "Torture Survivors," 2009.

Just Two People in a Room, Trying to Have a Body

1 *The Bhagavad Gita,* trans. Eknath Easwaran (Tomales, CA: Nilgiri Press, 2007), verse 6.20.

2 *The Yoga Sutras of Patanjali,* trans. Sri Swami Satchidananda (Buckingham, VA: Integral Yoga Publications, 1990), book 1, sutra 1.

My Road to Embodiment

1 Herman, *Trauma and Recovery,* 133.

A Feeling of Wholeness

1 Antonio R. Damasio, *The Feeling of What Happens: Body and Emotion in the Making of Consciousness* (Boston: Mariner, 2000), 28.

Flowing with Chaos

1 Chuang Tzu, *Basic Writings,* trans. Burton Watson (New York: Columbia University Press, 1964), 37–38.

2 Seng Ts'an, "Faith in Mind," A Buddhist Library, accessed February 29, 2020, http://www.abuddhistlibrary.com/Buddhism/C%20-%20Zen/Zen%20Poetry/Faith%20in%20Mind/Faith%20in%20Mind%20-%20By%20Seng%20T%27san.htm.

3 Herman, *Trauma and Recovery,* 133.

4 Gabor Maté, *In the Realm of Hungry Ghosts: Close Encounters with Addiction* (Berkeley, CA: North Atlantic Books, 2010).

5 David Emerson and Elizabeth Hopper, *Overcoming Trauma through Yoga* (Berkeley, CA: North Atlantic Books, 2011).

"I Was Able to Take Something Back"

1 Indra Devi, *Yoga for Americans* (1959; repr. Auckland, NZ: Pickle Partners Publishing, 2015).

2 Rowan Silverberg, "Trauma Center Trauma-Sensitive Yoga (TC-TSY) Peer Support Groups: An Adjunct Modality in a Feminist Approach to Trauma Treatment for Survivors of Sexual Violence" (PhD diss., Saybrook University, 2019), ProQuest (2366585926).

From Human Doing to Human Being

1 White Bison, *The Road to Wellbriety: In the Native American Way* (Colorado: White Bison, 2002).

2 *Collins Dictionary*, s.v. "being," accessed April 10, 2020, https://www.collinsdictionary.com/dictionary/english/being.

Roller Coasters

1 Fowler, "Visceral Sensory Neuroscience," 1505–1506.

2 Beate Herbert and Olga Pollatos, "The Body in the Mind: On the Relationship Between Interoception and Embodiment," *Topics in Cognitive Science* 4, no. 4 (2012): 692–704, https://doi.org/10.1111/j.1756-8765.2012.01189.x.

3 Bessel van der Kolk and Rita Fisler, "Dissociation and the Fragmentary Nature of Traumatic Memories: Overview and Exploratory Study," *Journal of Traumatic Stress* 8 no. 4 (1995): 505–525, https://doi.org/10.1002/jts.2490080402.

4 Kerry Ressler, "Protect Your Brain from Stress," Harvard Health Publishing, August 2018, http://www.health.harvard.edu/mind-and-mood/protect-your-brain-from-stress.

The Disconnected Self in Eating Disorders

1 Carolyn Costin and Joe Kelly, eds., *Yoga and Eating Disorders: Ancient Healing for Modern Illness* (New York: Routledge, 2016).

2 Hilde Bruch, *The Golden Cage: The Enigma of Anorexia Nervosa* (Cambridge, MA: Harvard University Press, 2001).

3 Katherine Dittmann and Marjorie Freedman. "Body Awareness, Eating Attitudes, and Spiritual Beliefs of Women Who Practice Yoga," *Eating Disorders* 17, no. 4 (2009): 273–292, https://doi.org/10.1080/10640260902991111.

4 Nayla M. Khoury, Jacqueline Lutz, and Zev Schuman-Olivier, "Interoception in Psychiatric Disorders: A Review of Randomized, Controlled Trials with Interoception-Based Interventions," *Harvard Review of Psychiatry* 26, no. 5 (2018): 250–263, https://doi.org/10.1097%2FHRP.0000000000000170.

5 Sena Bluemel, Dieter Menne, Gabriella Milos, and Oliver Goetze, "Relationship of Body Weight with Gastrointestinal Motor and Sensory Function: Studies in Anorexia Nervosa and Obesity," *BMC Gastroenterology* 17 no. 4 (2017): 1–11, https://doi.org/10.1186%2Fs12876-016-0560-y.

Be Myself; Be in My Self

1 Zadie Smith, *White Teeth* (New York: Vintage, 2000), 117.

2 Eli Clare, *Writing a Mosaic* (self-pub., 2016), https://eliclare.com/book-news/writing-a-mosaic.

3 "Requiem," from the musical *Dear Evan Hansen*, music and lyrics by Benji Pasek and Justin Paul (Milwaukee, WI: Hal Leonard, 2015).

4 Cheryl Strayed, *Tiny Beautiful Things: Advice on Life and Love from Dear Sugar* (New York: Vintage, 2012), 241–248.

Embers of Rage

1 Jennifer Inge West, "Moving to Heal: Women's Experience of Therapeutic Yoga after Complex Trauma" (PhD diss., Boston College, 2011), https://dlib.bc.edu/islandora/object/bc-ir:101480, p. 46.

Finding My Soul

1   David Emerson, lecture at Kripalu Center, Stockbridge, MA, October 28, 2013.
2   Bessel A. van der Kolk, Laura Stone, Jennifer West, Alison Rhodes, David Emerson, Michael Suvak, and Joseph Spinazzola, "Yoga as an Adjunctive Treatment for Posttraumatic Stress Disorder: A Randomized Controlled Trial," *Journal of Clinical Psychiatry* 75, no. 6 (2014), e559-e565.
3   Jon G. Allen, "Mentalizing in Practice," in *Handbook of Mentalization-Based Therapy*, ed. Jon G. Allen and Peter Fonagy (West Sussex, UK: Wiley, 2006), 3–30.

Relearning and Rewriting

1   Herman, *Trauma and Recovery*, 133.

INDEX

T

ACKNOWLEDGMENTS

——————————— Jenn Turner ———————————

I would like to thank my dear colleague Dave Emerson for putting faith in me early on in my career and supporting my development.

I am honored that each author for this book put their trust in me to work with them along this process—this book would not exist without you.

I am deeply grateful for all the teachings I have gained from my clients who have patiently allowed me to show up in vulnerability and imperfection.

I am especially grateful to S, who challenged me to write and speak with my voice and who taught me so much about healing.

I would like to thank the team at North Atlantic for their faith in this project and for their steady support along the way.

I would also like to thank my sister whose steadfast encouragement allowed me to step into this project.

——————————— Kirsten Voris ———————————

Gratitude to Jenn Turner for her thoughtful shepherding of this essay, the Tucson Writers' Table for helping me sit still once a week, and special love to Adam Hostetter for teaching me how to write about the bewildering and the joyful—by practicing alongside me.

To the Yoeme Kari Group Home residents and staff and the Pascua Yaqui Tribe Head Start summer program students and staff. Your curiosity and willingness inspired all of these words—and even more spiritual growth. Thank you.

—————————— Gwen Soffer ——————————

My deepest gratitude goes to the amazing Wellness Wednesday women who have taught me so much about the human capacity to love and heal. Your kindness, generosity, humor, and strength inspire us all.

—————————— Emily Lapolice ——————————

What an honor and privilege to be a part of this project and to be able to cultivate the distinct types of relationships, like the ones shared in this book, that are paramount to embodied trauma healing work. To Dave Emerson, Jenn Turner, and fellow colleagues at CFTE: finding my way to TCTSY nearly a decade ago has provided the integration, integrity, and scaffolding that have breathed life into my professional work and personal journey, enriching my sense of contribution and purpose, in ways I could have never imagined.

Thank you to my parents, husband, and family for always seeing and supporting me with fullness. Max and Elliot, I will forever offer you that same kind of space to grow into your authentic selves. Miriam, it has been an honor to fully "see" you; thank you for letting me share your story.

—————————— Elizabeth Ringler-Jayanthan ——————————

I want to acknowledge and thank all the courageous refugee women who have shared their stories with me and who choose hope despite facing unimaginable adversity.

—————————— Alexandra Cat ——————————

I'd like to dedicate my chapter to my Nan—the indomitable Ada Gold. You've been my rock for over fifty years. Thank you.

───────── Bailey Mead ─────────

As my story continues to unfold with each new season, I am filled with a renewed and ever-deepening sense of appreciation and gratitude for all of the beloved teachers and allies on my path, including my parents, Deborah and David; their partners, Tim and Cindy; my siblings, Erin, John, and Kimberly; my ancestors; my partner, Melissa Al-Azzawi; Jennifer Schatz; Calvin Graning; Jen Czach; John and Amy Hajec; Tameshia Bridges-Mansfield; Afeni Ngoze Hill; Susan Ryan; Barbara Kraft; Harriet Mall; Chuck Mallur; Jean Ogilve; Melissa Spamer; Elizabeth Wolff; Mia Henry; Marin Heinritz; Vanissar Tarakali; Kara Aubin; and countless others who told their stories and made mine possible. May my story be a light on someone else's way home.

───────── Jemma Moody ─────────

Heartfelt thanks to the remarkable and resilient children and families I have been privileged to walk alongside over the years. You are the reason I do the work. May you find peace and happiness.

───────── Eric Daishin McCabe ─────────

I'd like to thank my wife and families—both blood and spiritual—for continuing to open my eyes to notice both the beauty and ugliness of the world. I am indebted to so many teachers, too many to name, for my arrival in this moment.

───────── Rowan Silverberg ─────────

Activists never work alone; we depend on and inspire each other to keep on keeping on until the work is done. With deep gratitude and respect, I honor the contributions of my mother, Bea Silverberg; my dear friend and twin sister from another mother, T. Marion Beckerink; my brother, Mark Silverberg; and my son, Nehemiah Stark, to the fight for freedom and social justice for all.

Nicole Brown Faulknor

I would like to acknowledge God, first and foremost, in playing a protective and loving role in my healing journey. Alongside all the angels he's sent for me along the way through childhood friends, mentors, my therapist of almost ten years, my best friend and, most importantly, my children.

Kate O'Hara

Effie, writing this chapter with you was an honor. Through your quiet, reflective courage, I fully embraced how life's complexities can transform our humanity. With humility, gratitude, and a giant smile, thank you.

Rachael Getecha

To my husband, Mark, my forever and always, your unconditional love is my constant anchor. I am so grateful that I get to walk hand in hand with you on this journey. To my children, Kaya, Malik, and Malcolm, thank you for letting me see life through your unique perspectives every day. You are world changers. Continue to be brave and fearless in who you are. And to the One who holds the light, I thank You for always keeping me.

Cynthia Cameron

I would like to acknowledge the generosity of Jenn Turner and the editors of this book for including my experience (and for giving it clarity). I would also like to acknowledge the Center for Trauma and Embodiment, TCTSY program, which has provided a pathway for me to learn and use the wisdom of my experience in the service of others.

Simona Anselmetti

I would like to thank the amazing women that trusted and guided me in integrating my work with trauma and eating disorders and my passion for yoga: Sara Bertelli, Isabel Fernandez, and Francesca Cassia.

Thanks to Jenn Turner for the patience in editing my chapter and, last but not least, thanks to my family and colleagues that share in the intense work at Nutrimente Onlus.

—————————— Eviva Kahne ——————————

To my therapist, for all that was co-created through her guidance. To my family, for showing up in the newness. To all those I love and hold at the core of my heart, you know who you are.

—————————— Anna Kharaz ——————————

I'd like to first and foremost thank "Nicole": thank you for graciously sharing your trust with me and your story with us all. Your resilience, self-reflection, and overall badassery have been powerful teachers to me and it has been an honor to be alongside you on your healing journey. Thank you also to Meri Quinn for your literary skills, for your kind way of giving feedback, and for sharing your time. Thank you, Jenn, for bringing this book to life and helping share these stories of embodied healing.

—————————— Dallas Adams ——————————

I would like to acknowledge the folks that made this possible including my three co-authors, Dave Emerson and Jenn Turner, the founders and co-developers of Trauma Center Trauma Sensitive Yoga, and the patients and staff at the Menninger Clinic who have supported the delivery of TCTSY for the last five years. I would also like to acknowledge my wife and colleague, Lynn Quakenbush.

—————————— Jessica Rohr ——————————

I would like to acknowledge my authors for their kind, passionate, and empathic stance, as well as their enthusiasm for putting together a beautiful representation of how impactful TSY can be. I would especially like to acknowledge Kayla, who lent her voice to help others connect with the experience of working through TSY. Working with all of these individuals to adequately represent our experience took time, energy, and vulnerability, and I acknowledge all of us for being willing to give that to each other and whoever may benefit from our work.

———————————— Angelica Emery-Fertitta ————————

I have deep gratitude for the people and communities that allowed this work to be possible. I am specifically grateful to the young people I have had the opportunity to practice with as well as the CFTE for the opportunity to learn and grow in community. Finally, I am grateful for my parents, partner, and dear friends for their endless support over the last few years.

———————————— Christine Cork ————————————

I have such gratitude for the members of my TCTSY group. Thank you so much for being willing to be brave.

CONTRIBUTORS

Jenn Turner has been working in the field of trauma and yoga for over fifteen years. She is a co-founder and co-director of the Center for Trauma and Embodiment at Justice Resource Institute. In her role, she leads a global network of leaders in the field of embodiment and trauma. She leads trainings for other mental health care providers and embodiment practitioners throughout the US. Jenn also has a private psychotherapy practice in Boston, where she works to support survivors who are reclaiming and reintegrating their lives and bodies in the aftermath of trauma. To learn more, visit www.jenn-turner.com.

Kirsten Voris is a TCTSY facilitator and an essayist. Her work has been featured in journals such as *Superstition Review, Hippocampus,* and *Punctuate,* and the anthology *Expat Sofra: Culinary Tales of Foreign Women in Turkey* (Alfa). She is the co-creator of *The Trauma-Sensitive Yoga Deck for Kids* (North Atlantic Books) and lives in Tucson, Arizona.

Gwen Soffer is the wellness coordinator at Nationalities Service Center (www.nscphila.org) in Philadelphia, which serves individuals and families with refugee, asylum-seeking, and immigrant status. She has been developing, implementing, and facilitating trauma-sensitive wellness programming and trainings for over fifteen years. She coordinates onsite clinical and holistic wellness and leads a diverse team that includes a psychologist, art therapist, music therapist, movement therapist, acupuncturists, massage therapist, and reflexologist. Gwen facilitates trauma-sensitive yoga groups as part of a weekly program called Wellness Wednesday in addition to individual yoga sessions. She holds a master's in social work with trauma certificate from Widener University and is E-RYT certified through Yoga Alliance and TCTSY-F certified through the Center for Trauma and Embodiment at the Justice Resource Institute. She co-founded Enso yoga in Media, Pennsylvania, in 2007 as well as the Trauma-Informed Lens Yoga Certificate Program.

Emily Lapolice is an LICSW and TCTSY facilitator in private practice, specializing in complex trauma and perinatal mental health. She has worked in day-treatment, inpatient, school-based, and outpatient mental health settings in both New York City and Boston for the past fourteen years. Emily holds a bachelor's degree in psychology from Providence College and a master's degree in social work from New York University. Emily is also part of the training and supervisory faculty at the Center for Trauma and Embodiment at the Justice Resource Institute. She lives with her husband and two young boys in Arlington, Massachusetts. More information about Emily and her work can be found at www.iwtherapies.com.

Elizabeth Ringler-Jayanthan is a licensed social worker and a Trauma Center Trauma-Sensitive Yoga facilitator in Pittsburgh, where she works as a trauma therapist. She has worked primarily with survivors of forced migration including refugees, asylum seekers, and survivors of human trafficking. Elizabeth has also worked extensively with survivors of gender-based violence and currently works as a trauma therapist at a rape crisis center. She is a graduate of the Harvard Program in Refugee Trauma Global Mental Health Certificate program. Elizabeth is passionate about utilizing mind-body approaches in work with her clients, particularly mindfulness, trauma-sensitive yoga, and integrating nature into her work.

Alexandra Cat was originally schooled in Western approaches to psychology, philosophy, and neuroscience (Oxford and Sussex Universities). Alex shifted her emphasis from the intellectual to the physical in her late twenties, exploring body-based psychologies through her trainings and work in mountaineering/climbing, dance, and the Yoga Sutras. In both her individual and group work, Alex's interests are in early-life sexual assault and neglect, body dysmorphia, fantasy, escapism, and shame. Alex has a special interest in working with individuals who hold nonconforming sexuality or gender identities. Alex is in private practice through The Yoga Clinic (UK) and is a member of the teaching and training faculty for The Centre for Trauma and Embodiment.

Bailey Mead is a 500-hour registered yoga teacher and a TCTSY facilitator. She came to TCTSY through her own journey of seeking embodiment and healing through yoga. She experienced such a profound transformation that she trained as a yoga instructor in 2011 and went on to become certified as a TCTSY facilitator in order to make this practice accessible to others. Bailey believes it is each person's birthright to experience groundedness, wellness, peace, presence, and clarity in their body, and that it is never too late to seek this state of well-being. Her approach is grounded in a deep respect for each individual's experience and for the incredible gift of yoga Westerners have received from Indian culture. When she is not facilitating yoga, she also organizes global gatherings of social justice activists and works with her partner Melissa on creative projects in Kalamazoo, Michigan. Learn more at www.YogaForEmbodiment.com.

Jemma Moody is a social worker and TCTSY facilitator from Australia specializing in cross-cultural mental health social work. Jemma works with children, teens, and adults and has a background working with refugees and people seeking asylum as well as survivors of sexual and gender-based violence. Her work has involved developing and delivering a range of individual and group mental health and psychosocial programs internationally, including in Turkey, Greece, India, and Myanmar, with a focus on body-based interventions for mental health care and well-being. Jemma is particularly passionate about working alongside and supporting refugee and migrant communities globally in the field of mental health. In her decade-long experience working with displaced and culturally diverse populations, she has emphasized group work programs as tools for building community and belonging. Jemma is an advocate for accessibility and trauma-informed practice in mental health care and is passionate about the incorporation of somatic interventions to address and prevent mental health issues and improve well-being.

Eric Daishin McCabe is a priest in the Soto Zen school of Buddhism in Japan. With a keen interest in ecology and the world's faith traditions, he received his BA in religion and biology at Bucknell University in 1995. His early mentors were Professor John Grim and Mary Evelyn Tucker, with whom he studied interfaith dialogue with a special interest in Indigenous lifeways. He subsequently apprenticed with Patricia Dai-En Bennage Roshi of Mount Equity Zendo for fifteen years. During this time he trained at several Soto Zen monasteries in Japan as well as in France with the Venerable Thich Nhat Hanh. In 2013 he continued training in the art of spiritual direction and chaplaincy at Wellspan Hospital in Pennsylvania. He is recognized as an International Zen Teacher (Kokusaifukyoshi) by the Soto Shu. Daishin teaches world religions at Des Moines Area Community College and offers trauma-sensitive yoga at Broadlawns in Des Moines and at Central Iowa Psychological Services in Ames.

Rowan Silverberg, PhD, LMT, TCTSY-F, E-RYT 500, YACEP, has been working in the field of integrative health care for over thirty years. A graduate of Saybrook University's College of Integrative Medicine and Health Sciences, Rowan focused her doctoral research on trauma-sensitive yoga as an adjunct to clinical treatment for survivors of sexual violence. Rowan is certified as a trauma-sensitive yoga facilitator by the Trauma Center in Brookline, Massachusetts, and has led trauma-sensitive yoga support groups at the Cleveland Rape Crisis Center since 2016. Rowan is registered with the Yoga Alliance at the experienced yoga teacher (E-RYT 500) level and is a continuing education provider (YACEP). She has lectured on yoga to students at Case Western Reserve University's School of Medicine and Mandel School of Applied Social Sciences, is an adjunct faculty member at Cuyahoga Community College, and has designed and taught 200-hour yoga teacher training programs at yoga studios in the greater Cleveland area since 2004.

Nicole Brown Faulknor, founder of Wounds2Wings Psychotherapy, is a registered psychotherapist (qualifying) and child/youth counselor, a member of College of Registered Psychotherapists in Ontario and the Canadian Association for Psychodynamic Therapy, and a yoga instructor. With over eighteen years' experience, she has worked extensively with individuals and communities suffering from mental health problems, addictions, systemic poverty, and profiling to therapeutically improve relationships with government programs and services. Graduating from Mohawk College in 1988 with a diploma in child and youth counseling, Nicole received her bachelor's degree from the University of Waterloo in 2001 in social development studies with two certificates, general social work and a specialty in child abuse, including five-year master's equivalency diploma in 2018 from the Ontario Psychotherapy and Counseling Program, where she is currently a part-time instructor.

Kate O'Hara is a certified TCTSY facilitator (TCTSY-F) and a Yoga Alliance certified education provider (YACEP) with comprehensive experience facilitating movement and embodiment for people in recovery from complex trauma and substance use disorder. In private practice she partners with social service agencies to provide direct participant care as well as professional training workshops, supporting organizations in their transformation from trauma-informed systems to trauma-sensitive cultures. Since her thesis project work in industrial design, Kate has focused her attention on creating experiences where people have the opportunity to connect to themselves, others, and the wider world around them. Naturally curious, she's committed not only to professional development but also the rigorous exploration of self-study. For more information about Kate and her work in communities, you're welcome to visit www.thrivingtree.com.

Rachael Getecha is an E-RYT 200-hour yoga instructor, Yoga Alliance continuing education provider, certified Trauma Center Trauma-Sensitive Yoga (TCTSY) facilitator, and licensed 20-hour TCTSY trainer with the Center for Trauma and Embodiment. She works mostly in Idaho, Utah, and Nevada, and is a part of a cohort collaborating with a local wellness company to bring trauma-informed trainings to Eastern Africa. Inspired by her commitment to make yoga more accessible, in 2014 she started Amani Yoga, a mobile yoga company that offers trauma-sensitive yoga sessions and TCTSY trainings. She has experience teaching trauma-sensitive yoga with refugee populations, sexual abuse and assault survivors, youths, community trauma survivors, and those affected by PTSD and complex trauma. Rachael is passionate about collaborating with others to help build safer, more peaceful spaces within individuals, organizations, and communities through understanding trauma from a holistic lens. Rachael currently lives in Idaho, where there are more than just potatoes, with her phenomenal husband and three vivacious children.

Cynthia Cameron runs with her beloved dog and practices and teaches trauma-sensitive yoga in the Canadian prairies. She has a master's in intercultural communication, and she dabbles in teaching post-secondary communication and culture students, making art, and working out despite her years.

Simona Anselmetti is a psychologist-psychotherapist, TCTSY facilitator, EMDR accredited consultant, and Odaka yoga teacher. She's been working with trauma for twelve years, when she was trained in EMDR therapy. In the same period of her life she started to practice yoga, and in 2018 finally these two passions merged with the training in TCTSY. She is specialized in the treatment of eating disorders (ED) and has been working in a psychiatric unit for ED for fifteen years. Moreover, Simona is the co-founder of a nonprofit organization with the aim of preventing ED, also through yoga. She's been living in Milan, Italy, since university, and she loves traveling around the world, meeting people with different cultures, and working in groups with her colleagues. One of her major goals is to spread the importance of creating a trauma-informed environment in Italy as much as possible.

Eviva Kahne is a community organizer at the Boston Center for Independent Living. She works to engage people with disabilities in political spaces and to sustain member-led movements for accessible and affordable housing, health care, and public transportation. Eviva has a bachelor's degree in history, studied mass incarceration, and has a background in theatre. She is interested in engaging broadly in areas of social work and nonfiction writing, cultivating healing spaces, and investing in community.

Anna Kharaz is a licensed therapist and certified trauma-sensitive yoga facilitator. In addition to seeing clients for therapy and yoga, she serves as an adjunct faculty member and supervisor for the Center for Trauma and Embodiment at the Justice Resource Institute. She offers workshops and professional trainings across the United States and internationally to help health-care providers, educators, mental health professionals, yoga teachers, and bodyworkers better understand the impacts of trauma and implement trauma-informed practices in their work. Her approach to therapy, yoga, and education draws from a background in neuroscience, continued education in mental health and psychology, and a lifelong commitment to better understanding human suffering, health, and healing. You can learn more at www.wholehumancounseling.com.

Dallas Adams has been working with children, adolescents, and adults in the mental health field for over thirty years. In 2000, while living in Maine, he developed a yoga practice. Through this practice he learned he could experiment with life changes by first practicing them on the mat. In 2011 Dallas became a registered yoga teacher at the 200-hour level. During his mental health career, he became increasingly interested in complex trauma and its impact on people's lives. He completed the Trauma Center's

40-hour trauma-sensitive yoga course in 2013 and followed up with the Trauma Center's certification process in 2015. Since 2015 he's been teaching four group sessions of Trauma Center Trauma-Sensitive Yoga a week at The Menninger Clinic in Houston, plus TCTSY classes for individuals there. He is open to providing ongoing groups and individual sessions in other venues. You can contact him at dallasladams1@gmail.com.

Kayla Marzolino holds a bachelor's degree in business and now stays at home, raising her twin four-year-olds and her two-year-old. Recently she has pursued certification as a yoga instructor and is teaching yoga to people from all walks of life, from preschoolers to MMA fighters.

Jessica Rohr, PhD, is a licensed clinical psychologist at The Menninger Clinic and assistant professor at Baylor College of Medicine. Her clinical and research interests are related to improvement of women's mental health, especially when trauma is playing a role. She hopes to work to improve access to effective care.

Sonia Roschelli is a licensed clinical social worker and addictions counselor at The Menninger Clinic in Houston. She primarily works with young adults with co-occurring disorders. Sonia is a 200-hour registered yoga teacher, and she integrates approaches based in mindfulness, acceptance, mind-body, and self-compassion into her work with clients. She holds a BS in psychology from the University of Mary Washington and an MSW from George Mason University.

Angelica Emery-Fertitta, MSW, TCTSY-F, resides in Boston. Angelica has a passion for serving individuals and families managing experiences of disenfranchisement and mental health concerns. She is a graduate of Hampshire College and the Bridgewater State University School of Social Work. Angelica works to advance racial justice through her interventions and advocacy, as well as through the NASW-MA Racial Justice Council. She believes in the power of integrating a wide range of approaches into care and treatment, specifically for individuals who have experienced complex trauma. Angelica does this through yoga, peer support programming, creative interventions, and restorative practices with young people and their families in the greater Boston area.

Christine Cork is a licensed psychologist and Trauma Center Trauma-Sensitive Yoga facilitator (TCTSY-F) working at Cedar Centre Psychiatric Group in Cedar Rapids, Iowa. Christine specializes in working with adolescent and adult trauma survivors, anxiety, depression, and obsessive-compulsive symptoms. She has a special interest in working with individuals around issues of gender identity. Christine received her master's degree in community counseling from Georgia State University in 1993 and earned her psychology doctorate from the University of Northern Colorado in 2000. She has worked in community mental health, university counseling centers, and nonprofit social service agencies, and she currently sees adult and adolescent individuals. Christine offers a weekly group for adult trauma survivors incorporating TCTSY. More information about Christine and her current practice can be found at www.cedarcentrepsych.com/psychology.

About North Atlantic Books

North Atlantic Books (NAB) is an independent, nonprofit publisher committed to a bold exploration of the relationships between mind, body, spirit, and nature. Founded in 1974, NAB aims to nurture a holistic view of the arts, sciences, humanities, and healing. To make a donation or to learn more about our books, authors, events, and newsletter, please visit www.northatlanticbooks.com.

North Atlantic Books is the publishing arm of the Society for the Study of Native Arts and Sciences, a 501(c)(3) nonprofit educational organization that promotes cross-cultural perspectives linking scientific, social, and artistic fields. To learn how you can support us, please visit our website.